MCQs in
Gynecological Oncology

MCQs in
Gynecological Oncology

Editor

Bidhan Roy

MBBS MS DNB FGO PGDHHM

Reader - Instructor and Gyne Oncosurgeon
Department of Obstetrics and Gynecology
Armed Forces Medical College
Pune, Maharashtra, India

Co-Editor

Kamalika P Roy

MBBS DNB FICS PGDHHM PGDMLS

Maharashtra Institute of Medical Education
and Research (MIMER) Medical College
Pune, Maharashtra, India

Foreword
Aruna Menon

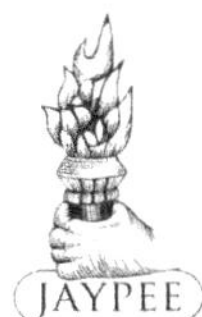

JAYPEE BROTHERS MEDICAL PUBLISHERS
The Health Sciences Publisher
New Delhi | London

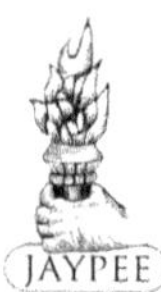

Jaypee Brothers Medical Publishers (P) Ltd

Headquarters
Jaypee Brothers Medical Publishers (P) Ltd
EMCA House, 23/23-B
Ansari Road, Daryaganj
New Delhi 110 002, India
Landline: +91-11-23272143
+91-11-23272703, +91-11-23282021
+91-11-23245672
Email: jaypee@jaypeebrothers.com

Overseas Office
J.P. Medical Ltd
83 Victoria Street, London
SW1H 0HW (UK)
Phone: +44 20 3170 8910
Email: info@jpmedpub.com

Corporate Office
Jaypee Brothers Medical Publishers (P) Ltd
4838/24, Ansari Road, Daryaganj
New Delhi 110 002, India
Phone: +91-11-43574357
Fax: +91-11-43574314
Email: jaypee@jaypeebrothers.com

EU GPSR Authorised Representative
Logos Europe, 9 rue Nicolas Poussin
17000, La Rochelle, France
Phone: +33 (0) 6 67 93 73 78
E-mail: Contact@logoseurope.eu

Website: www.jaypeebrothers.com
Website: www.jaypeedigital.com

© 2022, Jaypee Brothers Medical Publishers

Inquiries for bulk sales may be solicited at: jaypee@jaypeebrothers.com

MCQs in Gynecological Oncology

First Edition: 2022

ISBN: 978-93-5465-097-0

Dedicated to

Our Parents, Teachers, Students and Patients.

Reviewers of the Book

AC Kataki
Director and Professor
Department of Gynecologic Oncology
Dr B Borooah Cancer Institute
(An Unit of TMC, Mumbai)
Guwahati, Assam, India

Amita Maheshwari
Professor and Head
Division of Gynecologic Oncology
Tata Memorial Center
Mumbai, Maharashtra, India

Anitha Thomas
Associate Professor and HOD
Department of Gynecological Oncology
Christian Medical College
Vellore, Tamil Nadu, India

Bhagyalaxmi Nayak
Professor
Department of Gynecologic Oncology
Acharya Harihar Regional
Cancer Center
Cuttack, Odisha, India

BK Goyal
Consultant
Gynecologic Oncology and
Robotic Surgery
Armed Forces Medical Services
Pune, Maharashtra, India

Debabrata Barmon
Deputy Director (Academics)
Professor and In-Charge
Department of Gynecologic Oncology
Dr B Borooah Cancer Institute
(An Unit of TMC, Mumbai)
Guwahati, Assam, India

Gauri Gandhi
Professor
Department of Obstetrics and
Gynecology
Maulana Azad Medical College
New Delhi, India

Harshad Parasnis
Consultant Gynecologic Oncologist
Head of Gynecologic Oncology Unit
Bharati Vidyapeeth
Medical College, Pune
Visiting Gynecologic Oncologist at
BJGMC, Sassoon General Hospital
Pune, Maharashtra, India

Jaydip Bhaumik
Head of the Department
Gynecologic Oncology
Tata Memorial Center
Kolkata, West Bengal, India

Manash Biswas
Associate Director
Gyne Oncological Surgery
Specialist in HIPEC and Robotic Surgery
Max Institute of Cancer Care
Saket, New Delhi, India

Neerja Bhatla
Professor and HOD
Department of
Obstetrics and Gynecology
AIIMS, New Delhi, India

Rama Joshi
Director and HOD
Gynecologic Oncology and
Robotic Surgery
Fortis Memorial Research
Institute and Hospital
Gurugram, Haryana, India

Rupinder Sekhon
Senior Consultant and Chief
Gynecologic Oncology
Rajiv Gandhi Cancer Research Institute
New Delhi, India

Shalini Rajaram
Professor and Program Co-ordinator
MCh Gynecologic Oncology, AIIMS
Rishikesh, Uttarakhand, India

Foreword

I am extremely pleased to learn that the book titled *"MCQs in Gynecological Oncology"* happens to be the first of its kind! It is highly appreciable to see the hard work and sincerity with which the authors went through the latest guidelines and standard textbooks. The very thought of compiling MCQs requires extreme clarity and in-depth knowledge of the subject. I have witnessed the passion, perseverance and dedication of the authors while bringing out this book. I hope this book will certainly be very helpful for the postgraduate students who are preparing for further studies in Gynecological Oncology.

Best Wishes.

Aruna Menon
Professor and HOD
Department of Obstetrics and Gynecology
Armed Forces Medical College
Pune, Maharashtra, India

Preface

We are honored to author the book titled *"MCQs in Gynecological Oncology."* We have learnt a lot while compiling this book. It gave us an opportunity of understanding the subject better. Preparation for Gynecological or Surgical Oncology entrance examination requires a lot of hard work and proper guidance. As postgraduation offers only a limited exposure to Gyne Oncology, it becomes difficult for a student to find the exam oriented MCQs from the large volumes of standard textbooks. In Gynecological Oncology, there has always been a need of a concise, updated and conceptual study guide for the students. This book envisages such problems and helps mitigate them through an objective method of MCQs. Current MCQs are mostly based upon statistical facts but at times these quoted facts differ among the standard textbooks! Our endeavor has been to sincerely check the correctness of these facts and figures. We will be glad to get reviews by the readers and it will enrich us as authors. We humbly acknowledge our limitations and hence request to read our book along with the relevant chapters from the standard textbooks.

We are extremely thankful to the esteemed panelist of reviewers who guided and encouraged us to bring forth their ideas in this book. We are also thankful to the Jaypee Brothers Medical Publishers for their enriched values and their enormous trust in us for authoring this book. We are thankful to Mrs Kritika Dua, Senior Development Editor, for her sincerity and hard work in making this book. As we step forward, we bow with extreme gratitude to our parents and teachers.

Love to our daughters—Srinidhi and Sanaavi.

We hope that our students will be benefitted by this book.

Bidhan Roy
Kamalika P Roy

Acknowledgments

In humble and sincere acknowledgement of the golden opportunities for excellent training, career progression, personality enhancement, impeccable professionalism, love, honor and respect that is offered in the Armed Forces Medical Services.

"Sarve Santu Niramaya"
Jai Hind

Contents

Tumor Biology and Genetics in Gynecologic Oncology

1. Deoxyribonucleic acid (DNA) synthesis occurs in which phase of the cell cycle?

a. G1 phase
b. G2 phase
c. S phase
d. M phase

2. Cell division occurs in which phase of the cell cycle?

a. M phase
b. G1 phase
c. G2 phase
d. S phase

3. How many checkpoints are there in a cell cycle which can stop the cell cycle in case of any genotoxic insult?

a. 10
b. 08
c. 06
d. 04

4. Cell death pathways within a tumor include:

a. Apoptosis
b. Necrosis
c. Autophagy
d. All of the above

5. Which of the following illicit a brisk immune response?

a. Necrosis
b. Autophagy
c. Apoptosis
d. None of the above

6. *TP53* is a critical regulator of:

a. Autophagy
b. Necrosis
c. Apoptosis
d. None of the above

7. Telomerase is a critical regulator of:

a. Autophagy
b. Necrosis
c. Apoptosis
d. Cellular senescence

8. Two-step loss of tumor suppressor gene is evident in:

a. Hereditary cancer syndrome
b. Sporadic cancers
c. Both a and b
d. None of the above

9. p53 delays entry into which phase of the cell cycle?

a. G1 phase
b. G2 phase
c. S-phase
d. M-phase

10. "Guardian of the genome" is said to be:

a. Retinoblastoma (Rb) gene
b. TP53
c. TP16
d. TP27

11. As per the stem cell theory; the percentage of cancer stem cell in a malignant mass:

a. <0.5%
b. <1%
c. <5%
d. <10%

12. Molecular marker of cancer stem cells includes all, *except*:

a. CD133
b. CD117
c. CD24
d. CD100

13. For a cell to receive oxygen, it must be within how many μm from the capillary:

a. 10 μm
b. 100 μm
c. 20 μm
d. 200 μm

14. Angiogenesis is essential for a sustained malignant growth beyond:

a. 0.5 mm diameter
b. 5 mm diameter
c. 0.1 mm diameter
d. 1 mm diameter

15. "Warburg effect" in cancer biology means:

a. Aerobic glycolysis
b. Anaerobic glycolysis
c. Both a and b
d. None of the above

16. Not considered as a part of metastasis in cancer biology:

a. Angiogenesis
b. Invasion
c. Adhesions
d. Adaptations

17. ER and PR are classified as which types of biomarkers?

a. Diagnostic biomarker
b. Screening biomarker
c. Prognostic biomarker
d. Predictive biomarker

18. Use of poly ADP ribose polymerase (PARP) inhibitors in *BRCA* mutations is an example of:

a. Conditional lethality
b. Double lethality
c. Single lethality
d. Synthetic lethality

19. Common hereditary cancer syndromes include all, *except*:

a. Lynch syndrome
b. Familial adenomatous polyposis
c. Familial melanoma
d. Peutz–Jeghers syndrome

20. Mutations that affect familial cancer syndromes occur in what percentage in the general population:

    a. <1%   b. <3%
    c. <5%   d. <10%

21. **Most common extra-colonic malignancy in women with Lynch syndrome:**

    a. Ovarian cancer   b. Endometrial cancer
    c. Breast cancer   d. Renal cancer

22. **Most Lynch syndrome cases occur due to alterations in:**

    a. PMS1 and PMS2   b. MSH3 and MSH6
    c. MSH1 and MSH2   d. None of the above

23. **Percentage of endometrial cancer due to Lynch syndrome:**

    a. 3%   b. 5%
    c. 8%   d. 10%

24. **Type I endometrial cancers exhibit all, *except*:**

    a. TP53 mutations   b. PTEN mutations
    c. Microsatellite instability   d. β-catenin mutations

25. **Approximately, what percentage of ovarian cancer patients carry germline mutations of *BRCA1* and *BRCA2* genes?**

    a. 10%   b. 15%
    c. 20%   d. 25%

26. **_BRCA_ germline alterations are considered to be:**

    a. High-penetrance gene   b. Moderate-penetrance gene
    c. Low-penetrance gene   d. None of the above

27. **Use of oral contraceptive pills for 5 years in reproductive age reduces the risk of developing ovarian malignancy by:**

    a. 20%   b. 30%
    c. 40%   d. 50%

28. **Endometriosis has the potential of causing:**

    a. Endometrioid ovarian cancer   b. Clear cell ovarian cancer
    c. None of the above   d. Both a and b

29. **The phenomenon of platinum resistance in _BRCA_ related cancer ovary is due to:**

    a. Decreased sensitivity to platinum chemotherapy by *BRCA* mutations
    b. "Back mutations" in which the normal *BRCA1* or *BRCA2* sequence is restored
    c. "Double mutations" in which the normal *BRCA1* or *BRCA2* sequence is restored
    d. None of the above

30. **Polyadenosine diphosphate-ribose polymerase (PARP) inhibitor is associated with:**
   a. Synthetic lethality
   b. *BRCA*-related ovarian cancer treatment
   c. Benefits of non-*BRCA* mutations ovarian cancer treatment
   d. All of the above

31. **Mutations in ARID1A tumor suppressor gene is found in:**
   a. Endometrioid ovarian cancer
   b. Clear cell ovarian cancer
   c. Both a and b
   d. None of the above

32. **Mucinous ovarian cancer is associated with:**
   a. *KRAS* mutations
   b. *pTEN* mutations
   c. FOXL2 mutations
   d. ARID1A mutations

33. **Mutations in codon 134 of FOXL2 is associated with:**
   a. Endometrial ovarian cancer
   b. Clear cell ovarian cancer
   c. High grade serous ovarian cancer
   d. Adult granulosa cell ovarian cancer

34. **Mutations in *KRAS* gene is associated with all, *except*:**
   a. Borderline ovarian tumors
   b. Low grade serous ovarian tumors
   c. Mucinous ovarian cancers
   d. Endometrioid ovarian cancer

35. **Human papillomavirus (HPV) E7 oncoprotein inactivates:**
   a. TP53
   b. Retinoblastoma (Rb)
   c. TP16
   d. All of the above

36. **Human papillomavirus (HPV) E6 oncoprotein inactivates:**
   a. TP53
   b. Retinoblastoma (Rb)
   c. TP16
   d. None of the above

37. **Lower Anogenital Squamous Terminology (LAST) project incorporates which tumor suppressor gene to differentiate precancerous from normal lesions:**
   a. TP53
   b. Retinoblastoma (Rb)
   c. TP16
   d. TP52

38. **Mutations in *NLRP 7* gene is responsible for:**
   a. Recurrence in ovarian malignancy
   b. Recurrence in endometrial cancers
   c. Recurrence in molar pregnancy
   d. Recurrence in cervix cancer

39. Association of epidermal growth factor receptor (EGFR) and endometrial cancer are all, *except*:
   a. EGFR overexpressed in 43–67% of endometrial cancer
   b. Shortened disease free survival
   c. Shortened overall survival
   d. No change in overall survival

40. Genetic disorders associated with endometrial cancer:
   a. 10–15%
   b. 5–10%
   c. 3–5%
   d. 1–2%

41. Germline mutations found in Lynch syndrome (hereditary nonpolyposis colorectal cancer):
   a. *MLH1, MLH2, MSH6,* and *PMS2*
   b. *MLH2, MLH3, MLH4,* and *PMS1*
   c. *MLH3, MLH4, MLH6,* and *PMS2*
   d. *MLH2, MLH2, MLH6,* and *PMS2*

42. Lynch syndrome is associated with all, *except*:
   a. Increased risk of metachronous and synchronous cancers
   b. Broader spectrum of histology
   c. Increased incidence of lower uterine segment endometrial cancers
   d. Late onset of cancers than in general population

43. Amsterdam II criteria for Lynch syndrome include all, *except*:
   a. Three or more relatives have been diagnosed with Lynch syndrome-associated cancers
   b. Two affected relatives are in successive generations
   c. One affected relative is a first-degree relative of the other two
   d. One of the Lynch syndrome associated cancers must have been diagnosed before the age of 40 years

44. Risk reduction gynecological recommendations in Lynch syndrome includes:
   a. Endometrial biopsy every 1–2 years beginning at age 30–35 years
   b. Any abnormal uterine bleeding should be evaluated
   c. Chemoprevention with progestin-based contraception
   d. Risk reducing hysterectomy with salpingo-oophorectomy after completion of family
   e. All of the above

45. T-helper or inducer cells express:
   a. CD4 cell surface marker
   b. CD8
   c. CD10
   d. Both CD4 and CD8

46. T-suppressor or cytotoxic cells express:

a. CD4
b. CD8
c. Both CD4 and CD8
d. None of the above

47. CD4 Th1 is associated with:

a. Cellular immunity
b. Antibody response
c. Regulatory cells
d. All of the above

48. CD4 and TH2 is associated with:

a. Cellular immunity
b. Antibody response
c. Regulatory cells
d. All of the above

49. Treg cells are characterized by:

a. Suppress the activation and suppression of self-reactive lymphocytes
b. Express CD25
c. Express FOXP3
d. All of the above

50. TH1 is associated with:

a. IL-2 and IFN-Υ
b. IL-4 and IL-5
c. IL-6 and IL-10
d. Both b and c

51. TH2 is associated with:

a. IL-2 and IFN-Υ
b. IL-4 and IL-5
c. IL-6 and IL-10
d. Both b and c

52. *BRCA1* gene (hereditary breast ovarian cancer syndrome) is located in which chromosome?

a. 17q21
b. 13q12
c. 2q16
d. 17q13

53. *BRCA2* gene (hereditary breast ovarian cancer syndrome) is located in which chromosome?

a. 17q13
b. 13q12
c. 19q13
d. 17q21

54. Chromosomes implicated in Lynch syndrome:

a. 2p16
b. 7p22
c. 2p21
d. All of the above

55. Affected *PTEN* gene in Cowden syndrome is located in:

a. 10q23
b. 17q13
c. 17q21
d. 13q12

56. Affected *TP53* gene in Li–Fraumeni syndrome is located in:

a. 17q13
b. 10q23
c. 13q12
d. 17q13

57. Affected *STK11* gene in Peutz–Jeghers syndrome is located in:

   a. 19p13
   b. 17q13
   c. 10q23
   d. 13q12

58. *BRCA*-associated ovarian cancers are all, *except*:

   a. High-grade serous ovarian cancers
   b. Clear cell ovarian cancers
   c. Endometrioid ovarian cancers
   d. Mucinous ovarian cancers

59. Ideally (after child bearing) risk reducing salpingo-oophorectomy in *BRCA1* should be offered at the age of:

   a. 25–30 years
   b. 30–35 years
   c. 35–40 years
   d. 40–45 years

60. Ideally (after child bearing) risk reducing salpingo-oophorectomy in *BRCA2* should be offered at the age of:

   a. 25–30 years
   b. 30–35 years
   c. 35–40 years
   d. 40–45 years

61. Risk reduction percentage in *BRCA*-related gynecological cancers by risk reducing prophylactic salpingo-oophorectomy is estimated to be:

   a. 50%
   b. 40%
   c. 69%
   d. 96%

62. Percentage of serous tubal intraepithelial carcinoma (STIC) usually found in risk reducing salpingo-oophorectomy:

   a. 5–8%
   b. 0.9%
   c. 2.5%
   d. 10%

63. Hereditary pattern of autosomal dominant inheritance seen in ovarian cancer in:

   a. 20%
   b. 30%
   c. 10%
   d. 5%

64. Term used for growth and migration of tumor cells along host blood vessels:

   a. Vascular co-option
   b. Vascular attachments
   c. Intussusceptive angiogenesis
   d. None of the above

65. Prognosis of low-grade serous ovarian carcinoma depends upon:

   a. *BRAF*
   b. *KRAS*
   c. *ARID1A*
   d. *PTEN*

66. **Reed syndrome includes all, *except*:**
- a. Cutaneous piloleiomyomas
- b. Early-onset uterine leiomyomas
- c. Early-onset type II papillary renal cell cancer
- d. Autosomal recessive

67. **Clinical detection of a tumor is feasible when the minimum cell size is:**
- a. 10^9
- b. 10^{12}
- c. 10^{25}
- d. 10^{30}

68. **Tumor marker can detect a tumor when the minimum cell size is:**
- a. 10^9
- b. 10^{12}
- c. 10^{25}
- d. 10^{30}

69. **Mutations in BRCA is designated as a:**
- a. Predisposition markers
- b. Diagnostic markers
- c. Prognostic markers
- d. Predictive markers

70. **DICER 1 mutation is found in:**
- a. Epithelial ovarian cancer
- b. Sertoli-Leydig cell tumor
- c. Endometrioid ovarian tumor
- d. Granulosa cell tumor

ANSWERS KEY

1. c	2. a	3. d	4. d	5. a	6. c	7. d
8. c	9. c	10. b	11. b	12. d	13. b	14. d
15. a	16. d	17. d	18. d	19. c	20. a	21. b
22. c	23. a	24. a	25. a	26. a	27. d	28. d
29. a	30. d	31. c	32. a	33. d	34. d	35. b
36. a	37. c	38. c	39. d	40. c	41. a	42. d
43. d	44. e	45. a	46. b	47. a	48. b	49. d
50. a	51. d	52. a	53. b	54. d	55. a	56. a
57. a	58. d	59. c	60. d	61. d	62. a	63. a
64. a	65. b	66. d	67. b	68. a	69. a	70. b

NOTES: TUMOR BIOLOGY AND GENETICS IN GYNECOLOGICAL ONCOLOGY

- Hallmark of cancer is the dysregulation of normal cell cycle. The specific transitions in the cell cycle are controlled by the cyclin-dependent kinases (CDKs). Remember that there are four checkpoints in the cell cycle namely; G1/S, intra-S, G2/M, and at metaphase to anaphase. The cell cycle is divided into various sequential phases namely; protein synthesis in G1 phase, deoxyribonucleic acid (DNA) synthesis in S phase, cell growth in G2 phase, chromosomal segregation in mitosis, and cell separation in cytokinesis.
- All these three pathways namely autophagy, apoptosis, and necrosis may go on simultaneously in the tumor. Autophagy is a potentially reversible process in which a cell that is stressed "eats" itself. Apoptosis is an active energy-dependent and involves protein or DNA breakdown. *TP53* tumor suppressor gene is a critical regulator of apoptosis. Necrosis is not a well-regulated phenomenon and involves defects in osmoregulation and cellular fragmentation. This cellular fragments in necrosis can spill over into circulation and can cause an immune response.
- Cellular senescence is monitored by biologic clock and is due to the progressive shortening of repetitive DNA sequences (TTAGGG) called telomeres. Telomerase is RNA complex and is involved in chromosomal stabilization and in preventing recombination during mitosis. High telomerase activity is found in ovarian, endometrial, and cervical cancers.
- Gene encoding p53 tumor protein (TP53): TP53 is the most frequently mutated tumor suppressor gene in human cancer. It regulates genomic stability, cell cycle, apoptosis, and DNA protein repair mechanisms.
- Genetic "stem-cell-hit" theory of endometrial cancers is based upon the cancer stem cells. Cancer stem cells are considered to be a small subpopulation of tumor cells that have properties of tumorigenesis, potential for multiple lineages after differentiation, self-sustenance, and slow renewal by itself. Cancer stem cells are supposed to have been present in the transformation zone of the cervix, endometrial basal cells, and in the ovarian epithelial cells.
- Angiogenesis is an important character of cancer cell biology. Vascular endothelial growth factor VEGF-A, IL-8, beta-3 integrin, tyrosine kinase receptor EphA2, and matrix metalloproteinases act in angiogenesis for cancer growth. Bevacizumab is a VEGF-A receptor antagonist and is widely used in gynecological cancers. Normal cells use anaerobic glycolysis only in case of lack of oxygen but cancer cells use them even in presence of oxygen as their metabolic demand is more. This is known as "Warburg effect" or "aerobic glycolysis" of cancer biology. This task is collaborated in the cancer microenvironment by metabolic remodelling or reprogramming.

- Metastasis is a series of sequential steps like proliferation, angiogenesis, invasion, embolization, transportation, adherence, and extravasation. Genetic change in the cancer microenvironment directs cross-talk between the normal tissues and the cancer cells disregarding the antitumoral immune surveillance.
  (Please read about epithelial-to-mesenchymal transition in cancer biology that is associated with the aggressive variety of the epithelial ovarian cancer).
- Biomarker is an indicator of normal biological or pathological process or pharmacological responses to therapeutic interventions. It can be objectively evaluated and measured. Type 0 biomarkers relate to natural history of a disease and its clinical indices. Type 1 biomarkers relate to effects of therapeutic interventions. Examples of biomarkers are as follows:
  - Predictive biomarkers are used to identify those more or less likely to benefit from treatment due to its presence or absence
  - Predisposition biomarkers—DNA mismatch repair (MMR), *BRCA*
  - Screening biomarkers—PSA
  - Prognostic biomarkers-CA125
  - Diagnostic biomarkers—Immunohistochemical studies.
- Tumor markers are actually anything that can detect the presence of tumor in the body. Hence, it can be biochemical, hormonal, or imaging. Detection limit of usable tumor markers in clinical practice is in a tumor wherein the minimum size is of 10^9 cells. It is to be noted that a tumor is clinically detected when it attains a minimum size of 10^{12} cells.
- Now-a-days, "liquid biopsies" offer early detection and real-time monitoring of cancer progression. It includes measurements of circulating tumor cells, circulating tumor DNA, long noncoding RNA, circulating RNA, and tumor-derived exomes. Centrifuged supernatants of fine needle aspiration cytology (FNAC) samples have also been tried as liquid biopsy materials.
- Synthetic lethality is a genetic term used to describe a situation where a defect in each of the two pathways individually has no effect, but a defect in both pathways together results in cell death. *BRCA* mutated cells are sensitive to poly [ADP-ribose] polymerase 1 (PARP1) inhibition and go to apoptosis. PARP inhibitors (like olaparib, rucaparib, niraparib, talazoparib) block auto-PARylation and PARP1 dissociation from the single stranded breaks. In *BRCA 1* or *BRCA 2* mutated cells, these double-stranded breaks are not repaired and causing synthetic lethality.
- Henry Lynch syndrome [hereditary nonpolyposis colorectal cancer syndrome (HNPCC)] is defined as a hereditary predisposition to colorectal cancer and a wide range of other malignancies (endometrial, ovarian, and gastric cancer) as a result of germline mutations in mismatch repair (MMR). It is associated with mutations in *MSH2, MSH6, MLH1, PMS1,* and

PMS2. The risk of endometrial cancer is almost equal or more than that of colorectal cancer and, hence, precedes other cancers in this syndrome; thus, endometrial cancer is designated as the "sentinel cancer" in Lynch syndrome. The lifetime risk of ovarian cancer in Lynch syndrome is 6–12% and commonly occurs in between 42–49 years of age, usually in stage I or stage II and mostly of endometrioid or clear cell varieties. *MLH1* is the most affected one in case of endometrial cancers of Lynch syndrome.

- Please note that sixth edition of Barakat's Principles and Practice of Gynecologic Oncology (page 45) states that "the lifetime cancer risks in Lynch syndrome are about 70% for colon cancer, 40% for endometrial cancer, and 10% for ovarian cancer." But overall endometrial cancer due to Lynch syndrome is less.
- Favorable prognosis in endometrial cancers occur in association with mutations of polymerase epsilon (POLE) and high microsatellite instability (MSI-H).
- E6 and E7 are primary human papillomavirus (HPV) oncoproteins with numerous cellular targets. They are directly involved in cellular transformation of the HPV.
- E7 gene product binds with the retinoblastoma gene (pRb) and thus blocks the negative control of cell growth.
- E6 proteins binds the tumor suppressor protein p53 and also increases the telomerase activity.
  Please note: Four major steps in the development of cervical cancer are:
  1. Infection of the metaplastic epithelium of the TZ with the carcinogenic HPV.
  2. Viral persistence rather than clearance.
  3. Progression of persistently infected epithelium to cervical precancer.
  4. Invasion.
- Recurrent moles account for 2% of all hydatidiform moles. In a small number of cases, it is due to autosomal recessive familial recurrent hydatidiform mole syndrome. These are biparental in genetic origin.
- *BRCA* mutations:
  - Although ovarian cancer is mostly sporadic; but 10–14% of patients have a germline mutation in *BRCA1* or *BRCA2*. *BRCA* related hereditary ovarian cancers are generally associated with 10 years younger age at presentation than the nonhereditary ovarian cancers.
  - It is also to be noted that there is no significant family history of ovarian-related cancers in 44% of *BRCA* mutation positive women.
  - Specific *BRCA* mutations called founder effect mutations are clustered in certain ethnic groups like Ashkenazi Jewish descents.
  - It is recommended that *BRCA* mutation testing should be offered to all nonmucinous ovarian, fallopian tube, and primary peritoneal cancer patients. The overall survival of *BRCA* related ovarian cancers is better than the non-*BRCA* related ovarian cancers.

- – Ovarian cancers with germline or somatic *BRCA* mutations also respond better to platinum-based chemotherapy because the tumor cells are not able to repair intrastrand crosslinks formed by crosslinking platinum agents.
- Prophylactic salpingo-oophorectomy in premenopausal women has been reported to reduce the risk of developing subsequent breast cancer by 50–80%.
- KRAS stands for Kristen rat sarcoma.
- Reed syndrome is an autosomal dominant condition and is also known as hereditary leiomyomatosis and renal cell carcinoma (HLRCC).
- Common mutations in the cancer types:

Endometrial cancers	PTEN (favorable prognosis) & TP53 (poor prognosis)
High grade serous ovarian cancer	TP53, BRCA 1 & BRCA 2
Borderline serous ovarian cancer	KRAS
Ovarian clear cell carcinoma	ARID1A,
Endometroid ovarian cancer	ARID1A, PTEN, PIK3CA, PPP2RIA
Mucinous ovarian cancer	KRAS
Adult granulosa ovarian cancer	FOXL2

- ACOG and SGO recommendations for offering genetic risk assessment for hereditary breast and ovarian cancer syndrome:

20–25% chance of having inherited predisposition to breast and ovarian cancer
Women with personal history of both breast cancer and ovarian cancer
Women with ovarian cancer and a close relative with ovarian cancer or premenopausal breast cancer
Women with ovarian cancer of Ashkenazi Jewish ancestry
Women with breast cancer at age 50 years or younger and a close relative with ovarian cancer or male breast cancer at any age
Women with Ashkenazi Jewish ancestry in whom breast cancer was diagnosed at age 40 years or younger
Women with a close relative of a known BRCA1 & BRCA2 mutations
05%–10% chance of having inherited predisposition to breast and ovarian cancer
Women with breast cancer at age 40 years or younger
Women with ovarian cancer, primary peritoneal cancer or fallopian tube cancer of high- grade serous histology at any age
Women with bilateral breast cancer (particularly when the first case occurred <50 years of age)
Women with breast cancer at age 50 years or younger and a close relative with breast cancer at age 50 years or younger
Women with Ashkenazi Jewish ancestry with breast cancer at age 50 years or younger
Women with breast cancer at any age and two or more close relatives with breast cancer at any age (particularly when the first case occurred <50 years of age)
Unaffected women with a close relative who meets one of the previous criteria

- Risk-reduction recommendations by NCCN for carriers of BRCA 1 and BRCA 2 mutations:

Breast
Annual mammography and annual breast MRI starting by the age of 30 years
Risk-Reducing Salpingo-ophorectomy (RRSO) to reduce breast cancer risk between age 35 and 40 and when child bearing is complete
Consider chemoprevention with Tamoxifen or Letrozole
Consider risk reducing mastectomy
Ovary/Fallopian tube
RRSO to reduce ovarian and fallopian tube cancer risk between age 35 and 40 and when child bearing is complete
Consider chemoprevention with oral contraceptives
Consider ovarian cancer screening with six monthly transvaginal ultrasound and CA 125 from age 30-35 years until definitive risk-reduction with RRSO

- Risk-reduction recommendations by NCCN for women with Lynch Syndrome

Gastrointestinal
Colonoscopy every 1–2 years beginning at the age of 20–25 years
Consider upper GI endoscopy/capsule endoscopy every 2–3 years beginning at the age of 30-35 years
Consider chemoprevention with Aspirin or NSAIDs
Gynecologic
Patient should be aware that abnormal vaginal bleeding warrants evaluation
Consider screening with annual endometrial biopsy and transvaginal ultrasound beginning at age of 30 years
Consider chemoprevention with OCP or Progestins
Consider risk-reducing hysterectomy with bilateral salpingo-oophorectomy between age 35 and 40 and when child bearing is complete
Urologic
Consider annual urine analysis starting at the age of 25 to 30 years

- Molecular methods used in Oncology- (Better to have a basic idea of the following as it may be useful in multiple ways)
  - Real-time PCR (q-PCR), Allele-specific PCR (AS-PCR), Reverse transcriptase PCR (RT-PCR)
  - Fragment analysis
  - FISH
  - High-resolution melting curve analysis
  - Sanger sequencing
  - Pryosequencing
  - Single nucleotide extension assay (SNaPshot)
  - Next-generation sequencing (NGS)
  - Genomic microarray

Chemotherapy in Gynecological Oncology

1. The doubling time for germ cell tumor:

a. 20–40 days
b. 60–80 days
c. 100–120 days
d. 130–150 days

2. 1 cm malignant mass would have undergone:

a. 10 tumor doubling time
b. 20 tumor doubling time
c. 30 tumor doubling time
d. 40 tumor doubling time

3. The cell generation time means:

a. M phase to M phase
b. M phase to G1 phase
c. M phase to S phase
d. M phase to G2 phase

4. New deoxyribonucleic acid (DNA) replication occurs in:

a. G1 phase
b. S phase
c. G2 phase
d. M phase

5. Phase of cell division is:

a. G1 phase
b. S phase
c. G2 phase
d. M phase

6. Sanctuary sites in cancer biology means all, *except*:

a. Tumor is inaccessible to chemotherapeutic drugs
b. Drug concentration becomes less overactive for cell kill
c. Cerebrospinal fluid
d. Sites of cancer stem cells

7. Sanctuary sites in cancer biology means all, *except*:

a. Areas of tumor necrosis
b. Tumor cells with maximum growth fractions
c. Tumor cells with minimum growth fractions
d. Cerebrospinal fluid

8. Cockcroft–Gault equation for calculating carboplatin dose using estimated creatinine clearance or glomerular filtration rate (GFR) is based upon patient's, *except*:

a. Weight
b. Age
c. Height
d. Creatinine

9. **Recommended GFR in Calvert formula should not exceed:**

a. 125 mL/min

b. 150 mL/min

c. 140 mL/min

d. 100 mL/min

10. **Neutropenia can occur when absolute neutriphil count decreases below:**

a. 500 per mm^3

b. 1,000 per mm^3

c. 1,500 per mm^3

d. None of the above

11. **True about cisplatin and carboplatin are all, *except*:**

a. Cell cycle nonspecific bifunctional alkylating agents
b. Radiomimetic agents
c. Disrupts the DNA cross-linkages
d. G2 cell cycle arrest
e. S-phase cell cycle arrest

12. **Antitumor antibiotics include all, *except*:**

a. Actinomycin D

b. Bleomycin

c. Doxorubicin

d. Dacarbazine

13. **Antitumor antibiotics developed from fungi are all, *except*:**

a. Actinomycin D

b. Bleomycin

c. Mitomycin C

d. Dacarbazine

14. **Mechanism of action of cell-cycle nonspecific antitumor antibiotics include all, *except*:**

a. Intercalation into DNA base pairs
b. Formation of free radicals
c. Alteration of tumor cell membranes
d. Chelation of metal ions
e. Damages DNA intercross-linkages

15. **Paclitaxel acts by:**

a. Intercalation into DNA base pairs
b. Polymerization and stabilization of intracellular microtubules
c. Damages DNA intercross-linkages
d. All of the above

16. **Common side-effects of bevacizumab include all, *except*:**

a. Hypertension

b. Thromboembolism

c. Impaired wound healing

d. Risk of bowel perforation

e. Neuropathy

17. **Risk of teratogenic effects of chemotherapeutic agents are highest in:**

a. First trimester

b. Second trimester

c. Third trimester

d. Same in all trimester

18. **Antimetabolites include all, *except*:**

    a. Methotrexate   b. Gemcitabine

    c. 5-Fluorouracil   d. Paclitaxel

19. **Hypersensitivity reactions of Paclitaxel is due to:**

    a. Cremophor   b. Acrolein

    c. Adjuvant contents   d. None of the above

20. **Chemotherapeutic agents made from plant alkaloids include all, *except*:**

    a. Vincristine   b. Etoposide

    c. Docetaxel   d. Gemcitabine

21. **Mechanism of action of paclitaxel:**

    a. Disrupts the microtubular functions in a cell

    b. Inhibits the DNA

    c. Inhibits the ribonucleic acid (RNA)

    d. None of the above

22. **Which is not an epidermal growth factor receptor (EGFR)?**

    a. Trastuzumab   b. Pertuzumab

    c. Bevacizumab   d. None of the above

23. **Which is not an EGFR?**

    a. Gefitinib   b. Erlotinib

    c. Lapatinib   d. Pazopanib

24. **Antibody (Ab) against CA125 include:**

    a. Oregovomab   b. Abagovomab

    c. Both a and b   d. None of the above

25. **Dual EGFR and human EGFR-related receptor 2 (HER2) kinase Inhibitor:**

    a. Lapatinib   b. Cetuximab

    c. Trastuzumab   d. Gefitinib

26. **Bevacizumab targets:**

    a. Tyrosine kinases

    b. Epidermal growth factor receptors

    c. Poly (ADP-ribose) polymerase (PARP)

    d. Angiogenesis

27. **Which is not a PARP inhibitor?**

    a. Niraparib   b. Gefitinib

    c. Olaparib   d. Rucaparib

28. **Bevacizumab is a:**

a. VGEF-A Ab
b. VGEF-1 Ab
c. VGEF-2 Ab
d. VGEF-3 Ab

29. **Side-effects of bevacizumab include all, *except*:**

a. Hypertension
b. Thromboembolism
c. Impaired wound healing
d. Palmar-plantar erythrodysesthesia

30. **Trastuzumab is a monoclonal antibody that blocks:**

a. HER-2/neu receptor
b. EGFR
c. EGFR tyrosinase kinase
d. Dual EGFR/HER-2 neu kinase inhibitor

31. **Palmar-plantar erythrodysesthesia is a side-effect of:**

a. Liposomal doxorubicin
b. Docetaxel
c. Doxorubicin
d. Dactinomycin

32. **Tyrosine kinase inhibitors include all, *except*:**

a. Pazopanib
b. Cediranib
c. Sunitinib
d. Topotecan

33. **Topoisomerase inhibitors chemotherapeutic agent:**

a. Topotecan
b. Melphalan
c. Ifosfamide
d. Cisplatin

34. **Carboplatin include all, *except*:**

a. Conformational change in DNA
b. Bifunctional alkylating like agent
c. Highly neurotoxic
d. More hematopoietic toxicity

35. **Antitumor antibiotics include all, *except*:**

a. Dactinomycin
b. Doxorubicin
c. Liposomal doxorubicin
d. Docetaxel

36. **Second malignancies are associated with all, *except*:**

a. Melphalan
b. Etoposide
c. Procarbazine
d. Paclitaxel

37. **Chemotherapeutic agents with highest gonadal toxicity:**

a. Vinca alkaloids
b. Antimetabolites
c. Alkylating agents
d. Antitumor antibiotics

38. Cardiac toxicity is usually seen with all, *except*:

a. Doxorubicin
b. Busulfan
c. Trastuzumab
d. Cyclophosphamide

39. True about neurotoxicity of cisplatin include all, *except*:

a. Progressive peripheral neuropathy
b. Delayed peripheral neuropathy
c. Sensory neuropathy
d. Motor neuropathy

40. Endocardial fibrosis is a side effect of:

a. Busulfan
b. Mitomycin C
c. Methotrexate
d. All of the above

41. Myocardial fibrosis is a side effect of:

a. Busulfan
b. Mitomycin C
c. Methotrexate
d. All the above

42. Hepatic fibrosis is a side effect of:

a. Busulfan
b. Mitomycin
c. Methotrexate
d. All the above

43. Severe cardiomyopathy can be a side effect of:

a. Doxorubicin
b. Docetaxel
c. Bevacizumab
d. Trastuzumab

44. Nephrotoxic side effect of cisplatin is by:

a. Damage of renal tubular cells
b. Oliguric renal failure
c. Interstitial nephritis
d. All the above

45. Nephrotoxic side effect of methotrexate is by:

a. Damage of renal tubular cells
b. Oliguric renal failure
c. Interstitial nephritis
d. All of the above

46. Neuropathy of vincristine first affects:

a. Loss of deep tendon reflex and distal paresthesia
b. Postural hypotension
c. Urinary retention
d. Facial palsy

47. Neuropathy is a side effect of:

a. Vinca alkaloids
b. Cisplatin
c. Paclitaxel
d. All of the above

48. Skin necrosis by extravasation is a side effect of:

a. Vincristine
b. Actinomycin D
c. Doxorubicin
d. All of the above

49. **Interstitial pneumonitis is a side effect of:**

a. Bleomycin
b. Gemcitabine
c. Nitrosoureas
d. All of the above

50. **Radiation recall dermatological reactions is seen with:**

a. Bleomycin
b. Actinomycin D
c. Methotrexate
d. Doxorubicin

51. **Drugs causing severe alopecia include all, *except*:**

a. Carboplatin
b. Paclitaxel
c. Docetaxel
d. Cyclophosphamide

52. **As per RECIST criteria: 30% reduction in the sum of diameters of all target measurable lesions:**

a. Complete response
b. Partial response
c. Progressive disease
d. Stable disease

53. **RECIST stands for:**

a. Response Evaluation Criteria in Solid Tumors
b. Response Estimation and Control in Solid Tumors
c. Recount Evaluation Criteria in Solid Tumors
d. Response Endorsement and Control in Solid Tumors

54. **Delayed bone marrow suppression is seen with:**

a. Carboplatin
b. Paclitaxel
c. Cisplatin
d. Mitomycin C

55. **Drug interactions causing maximum clinical benefit:**

a. Additive effect
b. Synergistic effect
c. Antagonistic effect
d. Multiplication effect

56. **In dose dense chemotherapy:**

a. Increasing frequency of chemotherapy
b. Increasing dose of chemotherapy
c. Increasing both dose and frequency of chemotherapy
d. None of the above

57. **Drugs acting in the mitotic phase (M) of the cell cycle include all, *except*:**

a. Paclitaxel
b. Vincristine
c. Vinblastine
d. Doxorubicin

58. **Doxorubicin acts upon which phase of the cell cycle?**

a. Mitotic (M) phase
b. Postmitotic (G1) phase
c. Early synthetic phase
d. Late synthetic phase

59. **Drugs acting in the postmitotic phase of the cell cycle:**

a. Actinomycin D
b. Methotrexate
c. 5-Fluorouracil
d. Hydroxyurea

60. **Drugs acting in the early synthetic phase of the cell cycle include all,** *except:*

a. Methotrexate
b. 5-Fluorouracil
c. Hydroxyurea
d. Actinomycin D

61. **Drugs acting in the postsynthetic phase of the cell cycle include all,** *except:*

a. Carboplatin
b. Cisplatin
c. Etoposide
d. Paclitaxel

62. **Tumors grow in a sigmoidal growth pattern is known by:**

a. Gompertzian growth theory
b. Skipper's cell kill theory
c. Goldie–Coldman theory
d. Norton–Simon theory

63. **Chemotherapeutic agents work by first order kinetics is given by:**

a. Gompertzian growth theory
b. Skipper's cell kill theory
c. Goldie–Coldman theory
d. Norton–Simon theory

64. **Sequential use of chemotherapeutic drugs to produce maximal effects and minimizing resistance is given by:**

a. Norton–Simon theory
b. Goldie–Coldman theory
c. Skipper's cell kill theory
d. Gompertzian growth theory

65. **Increase treatment efficacy of chemotherapeutic drugs with the use of optimal dose levels:**

a. Norton–Simon theory
b. Goldie–Coldman theory
c. Skipper's cell kill theory
d. Gompertzian growth theory

66. **Current use of bevacizumab in ovarian cancer includes:**

a. Combination therapy
b. Maintenance therapy
c. Platinum resistant ovarian cancer
d. All of the above

ANSWERS KEY

1. a	2. c	3. a	4. b	5. d	6. d	7. c.
8. c	9. a	10. a	11. e	12. d	13. d	14. e
15. b	16. e	17. a	18. d	19. a	20. d	21. a
22. d	23. d	24. c	25. a	26. d	27. b	28. a
29. d	30. a	31. a	32. d	33. a	34. c	35. d
36. d	37. c	38. d	39. d	40. a	41. b	42. c
43. a	44. a	45. b	46. a	47. d	48. d	49. d
50. d	51. a	52. a	53. a	54. c	55. b	56. a
57. d	58. d	59. a	60. d	61. d	62. a	63. b
64. b	65. a	66. d				

NOTES: CHEMOTHERAPY IN GYNECOLOGICAL ONCOLOGY

- Response evaluation criteria in solid tumors:
  - The target lesions are those which are suitable for repeated radiological assessment and depends upon their size [lesions with longest diameter (LD)].
  - *Complete response (CR)*: Disappearance of all target lesions.
  - *Partial response (PR)*: At least a 30% decrease in the sum of the LD of target lesions, taking reference of the baseline sum of LD.
  - *Progressive disease (PD)*: At least a 20% increase in the sum of the LD of target lesions, taking as reference the smallest sum of LD recorded since the treatment started or the appearance of one or more new lesions.
  - *Stable disease (SD)*: Neither sufficient shrinkage to qualify for PR nor sufficient increase to qualify for PD, taking as reference the smallest sum of LD since the treatment started.
  - Limitations include the inability to measure the extent of response in sites with unmeasurable tumor (pleural, ascitic, bone and leptomeningeal disease).
- Hypothesis in chemotherapy:
  - *Skipper's hypothesis (log kill hypothesis)*: If the tumor were treated at the level of micro metastases rather than larger volume tumors, it was more

likely that the treatment would be effective. Chemotherapeutic agents work by first-order kinetics and that they kill a constant fraction of cells rather than a constant number of cells. It also extrapolates the need for intermittent courses of chemotherapy to achieve the magnitude of cell kill necessary to produce tumor regression and cure. It also provides a rationale for multiple-drug or combination chemotherapy.

- *Goldie–Coldman hypothesis*: Spontaneous mutation to a drug-resistant phenotype occurs in rapidly growing malignant tumors at variable rate. This model predicts that alternating cycles of treatment should be superior to the sequential use of particular agents because sequential use of antineoplastic drugs would allow for the development and regrowth of a doubly resistant line.
- *Norton–Simon hypothesis*: The efficacy of treatment for tumors exhibiting sensitivity to particular chemotherapeutic agents will be enhanced if single agents, or in combination regimes, are delivered at their optimal dose levels in a so-called dose-dense manner, rather than as alternating regimes. It focuses on the rapid administration of as many active agents as possible and frequent modification of dose levels because of overlapping side effects of the chemotherapeutic agents.
- Dose-dense and dose-fractionated chemotherapy may be more active than the same treatment given every 3 week. The antiangiogenic effect of weekly metronomic chemotherapeutic agent decreases the accelerated repopulation of cancer cells between cycles and also reduces the acquisition of drug resistance.

- Hyperthermic intraperitoneal chemotherapy (HIPEC) is a highly concentrated and heated chemotherapy treatment that is delivered directly to the abdomen during surgery. This procedure is used to treat tumors in the peritoneal lining of the abdomen that results from ovarian, gastric, colon, appendix tumors, mesothelioma, and other types of cancers.

- Pressurized intraperitoneal aerosol chemotherapy (PIPAC) is a procedure where aerosolized chemotherapy is directly injected into abdomen via a high-pressure injector.

- *Metronomic therapy:* Repeated administration of chemotherapeutic drugs at low doses frequently and without any prolonged drug free period. The aim is to avoid adverse side-effects of chemotherapeutic agents which causes disruption of chemotherapy treatment. It uses biological optimised dose instead of maximum tolerated dose and preferably by oral administration. It acts by multi-targeted mechanism like anti-angiogenesis mechanism, enhancing immune mechanism and by inducing tumor dormancy. Use of metronomic therapy may lead to development of potential drug resistance. Example of metronomic therapy are use of Cyclophosphamide and Methotrexate.

Radiation Therapy in Gynecological Oncology

1. **Radiation causes cell death by:**
   - a. Mitotic cell death
   - b. Programmed cell death
   - c. Both a and b
   - d. None of the above

2. **Most common cause of cell death by radiation is:**
   - a. Mitotic cell death
   - b. Apoptosis
   - c. Necrosis
   - d. Autophagy

3. **"Dose-rate" effect is efficiently used in case of:**
   - a. High dose rate (HDR) brachytherapy
   - b. Interstitial brachytherapy
   - c. Stereotactic body radiation therapy
   - d. Intensity-modulated radiation therapy
     (dose-rate effect is also used for LDR brachytherapy)

4. **The four 'R' of radiobiology includes:**
   - a. Repair-repopulation-redistribution-reoxygenation
   - b. Repopulation-regeneration-repair-reoxygenation
   - c. Recycling-repair-regeneration-reoxygenation
   - d. Recycling-regeneration-repair-repopulation

5. **In radiation therapy-altered fraction protocols require a minimum interval between treatments for repair of accumulated sublethal injury:**
   - a. 2–4 hours
   - b. 4–6 hours
   - c. 6–8 hours
   - d. 8–10 hours

6. **Cells are most radiation sensitive in which phase of cell cycle?**
   - a. G2 and mitotic phase
   - b. S phase
   - c. G1 phase
   - d. All of the above

7. **Cells are most radiation resistant in which phase of cell cycle?**
   - a. G1 and S phase
   - b. G2 and S phase
   - c. Mitosis and S phase
   - d. None of the above

8. **The most effective radiation sensitizer is:**
   - a. Oxygen
   - b. Chemotherapy
   - c. Drugs
   - d. Temperature

9. **What is the recommended hemoglobin (Hb) level at the time of radiation?**

a. 8 gm/dL

b. 10 gm/dL

c. 12 gm/dL

d. 14 gm/dL

10. **Ovarian failure occurs at what dose of radiation in an adult?**

a. 10 Gy

b. 20 Gy

c. 30 Gy

d. 40 Gy

11. **Rectum and urinary bladder tolerate a dose of radiation without serious side effects:**

a. 45–50 Gy

b. 50–60 Gy

c. 60–70 Gy

d. 20–30 Gy

12. **Transient depletion of bone marrow elements occurs at a minimum dose of what radiation?**

a. 5–10 Gy

b. 10–15 Gy

c. 15–20 Gy

d. 20–25 Gy

13. **In hyper-fractionated radiation strategy; all are true, *except*:**

a. Dose per fraction is reduced

b. Number of fractions and total dose are increased

c. Overall treatment time is relatively unchanged

d. Dose per fraction is increased

14. **In accelerated radiation strategy; all are true, *except*:**

a. Dose per radiation is unchanged

b. Total dose is unchanged or decreased

c. Overall treatment duration is reduced

d. Dose per fraction is increased

15. **In hypo-fractioned radiation strategy; all are true, *except*:**

a. Dose per fraction is increased

b. Number of fractions and total dose are reduced

c. Overall treatment time is decreased

d. Dose per fraction is decreased

16. **1 Gray (Gy) is equal to:**

a. 10 rad

b. 100 rad

c. 1000 rad

d. None of the above

17. **Relative biologic effectiveness is defined as the ratio between a test radiation dose and:**

a. The dose of 100 KV X-rays needed to produce a specific biologic effect

b. The dose of 150 KV X-rays needed to produce a specific biologic effect
c. The dose of 200 KV X-rays needed to produce a specific biologic effect
d. The dose of 250 KV X-rays needed to produce a specific biologic effect

18. **Reference points A used in Manchester system include the following:**

a. Point A is 2 cm lateral and 2 cm superior to external cervical orifice (os) in the plane of the implant
b. Point B is 3 cm lateral to point A
c. Point A is 2 cm lateral and 2 cm superior to internal cervical os in the plane of implant
d. Doses from intracavitary and external beam radiation therapy may not be biologically equivalent

19. **Reference point B used in Manchester system:**

a. Point B is 5 cm from midline at the level of point A
b. Corresponds to obturator lymph nodes
c. Corresponds to the crossing of ureter and uterine artery
d. Radiation doses are titrated differently for point A and point B

20. **Late radiation complications occur after how many days of treatment?**

a. 60 days
b. 90 days
c. 120 days
d. 180 days

21. **Bragg's peak principle is shown by:**

a. Photons
b. Protons
c. Electrons
d. Neutrons

22. **Compton scatter principle is seen in case of:**

a. Photons
b. Protons
c. Alpha particles
d. Neutrons

23. **True in radiation therapy include:**

a. Dose of radiation from a source to any point in space varies according to the inverse of the square of the distance from the source to the point
b. Dose of radiation from a source to any point in space varies according to the square of the distance from the source to the point
c. Dose of radiation from a source to any point in space is directly proportional to the distance from the source to the point
d. Dose of radiation from a source to any point in space varies according to the inverse of the cube of the distance from the source to the point

24. Treatment strategies in radiation oncology for overcoming radioresistance of hypoxic cells include all, *except*:

a. Hyperbaric oxygenation
b. Misonidazole
c. Low linear energy type of radiation
d. Packed RBC transfusion

25. No observed adverse effect level (NOAEL) in case of radiation therapy effect during pregnancy is:

a. 1 rad
b. 2 rad
c. 3 rad
d. 5 rad

ANSWERS KEY

1. c	2. a	3. b	4. a	5. b	6. a	7. a
8. a	9. a	10. b	11. a	12. b	13. d	14. d
15. d	16. b	17. d	18. c	19. c	20. b	21. b
22. a	23. a	24. c	25. d			

NOTES: RADIATION ONCOLOGY IN GYNECOLOGICAL ONCOLOGY

- Elements of ionizing radiation include X-rays, gamma-rays, electrons, protons, neutrons, and alpha particles:
  - X-rays and gamma-rays (they are designated as photons) interact with matter by:
    - Photoelectric effect is proportional Z^3
    - Compton scatter depends upon the density of the absorbing materials. The photon particles interact with the outer shell electrons
    - Pair production absorption is related to Z^2 (Z is the atomic number of the absorbing materials).
  - *Electrons:* Acts on superficial targets without any significant effect in the underlying tissues. They are very light particles.
  - *Protons:* They are positively charged heavier particles and deposits maximum of their energy at a depth as per the *Bragg peak principle*. It is ideal for conformal therapy due to no exit dose.
  - *Neutrons:* They are neutral particles and tend to deposit most of their energy in a single intranuclear event. They deposit heavy energy at tissues and are associated with high complications rate.

- *Alpha particles:* Less clinical applications.
- Unit of radiation dose measurement is Gray (Gy). Absorbed dose is a measure of the energy deposited by radiation source in the target material (1 Gy = 1 Joule/kg of absorbing material) (1 rad = 1 cGy and 1 Gy = 100 rad).
- Rate of decay of a sample of radioactive material is measured in curies (Ci) and Becquerel. 1 Ci = 3.7×10^{10} disintegrations per second and 1 mCi = 10^{-3} Ci.
- Radioactive isotopes use in radiation biology: ^{226}Ra, ^{222}Rn, ^{137}Cs, ^{192}Ir, ^{60}Co, ^{125}I, ^{131}CS, ^{90}Sr, ^{169}Yb, ^{145}Sm, and ^{241}Am.
- Radiation targets deoxyribonucleic acid (DNA) damage—causes both mitotic cell death and programmed cell death (apoptosis). Deoxyribonucleic acid breaks, apoptosis cascade activation, release of cellular debris, and stimulation of cytokines (calreticulin) and causes an imbalance between regulatory and nonregulatory functions of T cells.
- *Cell survival curves:* Graphical representations of the effects of ionizing radiation on the survival of cell populations in vitro:
  - Multitarget model (all sensitive targets to hit for killing cells).
  - Linear quadratic model (one is proportional to the dose and the other component is proportional to the dose).
  - *Dose-rate effect:* Decreased dose-rate gives the cells a greater opportunity to repair sublethal injury during the exposure.
  - Biologic effects of radiation dose include dose, fraction size, interfraction interval and time over which the dose is given.
  - Biologically effective dose compares the various fractionation schedules.
  - Dose rate effect implies that the cells have a greater opportunity to repair sublethal injury during the exposure of an increasing dose of radiation.
  - Therapeutic ratio means the difference between tumor control and normal tissue complications, depends upon the fractionation of the dose and sensitivity of the dose.
- Radiation therapy (RT) is delivered by external beam radiation (EBRT), brachytherapy [low dose rate (LDR)— Ra and Cs and HDR—Ir], and as radioactive solutions.
- EBRT = external beam radiation therapy, GTV = gross target volume, CTV = clinical target volume, ITV = internal target volume, IMRT = intensity-modulated radiation therapy, LDR brachytherapy = low dose rate brachytherapy, HDR brachytherapy = high dose rate brachytherapy.
- The four "R" of radiobiology are repair, repopulation, redistribution and reoxygenation.
- Repair:
  - Fractionated irradiation permits greater recovery of sublethal injury during the treatment.

- Higher total dose of radiation is required to achieve a given biologic effect when the total dose is divided into smaller fractions.
- Repopulation:
  - Cell proliferation trigger that occurs during delivery of a course of radiation treatment.
  - Accelerated repopulation may increase the detrimental effect of treatment delays and may influence the effectiveness of sequential multimodality treatments.
- Redistribution:
  - Cells are sensitive to radiation in late G2 phase and most resistant in mid to late S and early G1 phases.
  - Redistribution to more sensitive phases of the cell cycle.
- Reoxygenation:
  - Sensitivity of fully-oxygenated cells to sparsely ionizing radiation is 3 times that of cells irradiated under anoxic conditions.
  - The ratio between the dose needed to achieve a given level of cell death under oxygenated versus hypoxic conditions is referred to as the oxygen enhancement ratio.
- Linear-energy transfer is the rate of deposition of energy along the path of a radiation beam, depends upon cell death magnitude and repairable cell populations:
  - Low linear energy transfer by X-rays, gamma-rays, protons, and electrons.
  - High linear energy transfer by neutrons, alpha particles, and carbon ions. There is no repairable injury, magnitude of cell death from a given radiation dose is greater and oxygen enhancement ratio is diminished.
  - Relative biologic effectiveness is defined as the ratio between the test radiation dose and the dose of 250-kV X-rays needed to produce a specific effect.
  - Temperature can modify the effect of ionizing radiation. Temperature of 42–43°C sensitize cells to radiation.
  - Dose of radiation from a source to any point in space varies according to the inverse of the square of the distance from the source to the point (inverse square law).
- Treatment strategies for overcoming radio-resistance of hypoxic cells are hyperbaric oxygen, red cell transfusion, hypoxic cell sensitizer drugs (misonidazole), and high linear energy transfer radiation.
- Adverse effects of radiation exposure:
  - Acute reactions to radiation include diarrhea (mucosal denudation) and radiation dermatitis.
  - Late reactions of radiations are due to damage to vascular stroma and proliferating stem cells. There is subsequent fibrosis and followed by loss of function.
  - Deterministic effects: No observed adverse effect level (NOAEL)—0.05 Gy or 5 rad; Gross fetal malformations—0.2 Gy or 20 rad.

- – Stochastic effects:
    - – Unpredictable oncogenic or mutagenic effects
    - – Mental retardation (mostly when 8–15 weeks POG 4% in 10 rads to 60% in 150 rads). Please note: X-ray dosimetry tables (CT scan pelvis: 0.25–1.5 rads, CXR: 0.0002–0.0007 rads).
- • Various fraction doses of radiation:

Fractionated radiation therapy (RT)	Dose per fraction	Number of fractions	Total dose	Overall treatment time	Uses
Hyperfrac-tionation	Reduced	Increased	Increased	Unchanged	Avoid side-effects of higher dose
Accelerated fractionation	Unchanged	Increased	Unchanged or decreased	Reduced	Does not reduce late effects but increases the acute effects
Hypofrac-tionation	Increased	Reduced	Reduced	Reduced	Palliative RT Stereotactic RT

- • Site specific maximum tolerable dose of radiation:

Site/organ specific	Maximum tolerable dose
Uterus	It can tolerate up to 100 Gy but at 50 Gy it loses the capacity of carrying pregnancy
Ovary	20 Gy depends upon the age of the patient
Vagina	40 Gy causes loses of vaginal elasticity
Small intestine	30 Gy
Rectum	45–50 Gy
Bladder and ureter	45–50 Gy and 85–90 Gy
Kidney	18–22 Gy
Liver	30 Gy
Bone marrow	Transient depletion at 10–15 Gy and permanent depletion at 30–40 Gy
Spinal cord	60 Gy

- • External beam radiation treatment planning:

Anterior-posterior border	Inferior: Mid-pubis or 3–4 cm from the most distal point of the disease in the cervix or vagina	Superior: L4–L5 interface	Lateral: 1.5–2 cm lateral to pelvic nodes or 1 cm lateral to the margin in bony pelvic wall

Contd...

Contd...

Lateral border	Inferior and superior: Same as above	Anterior: 1.5–2 cm anterior to iliac nodes covering obturator nodes should include the entire uterus	Posterior: 1.5–2 cm posterior to the iliac nodes with the posterior margin at S1–S3

Point A: A point 2 cm lateral and 2 cm superior to the external cervical os in the plane of the implant
Point B: A point 3 cm lateral to point A
Four fields are generally preferred

- Types of brachytherapy (LDR, HDR, and PDR):

LDR	*HDR*	*PDR*
72–96 hours	Minutes to hours	Intermittent pulses
Caesium	Iridium In OPD basis Heavily shield room is required and should maintain high quality standard	

(HDR: high dose rate; LDR: low dose rate; PDR: pulsed dose rate)

- Clinical applications of RT in cancer cervix:

Definitive surgery: Stage IA (fertility preserving surgery), IB1, IB2, and II A1; definitive concurrent RT: Stage IB3, II A2-IV A, unfit for sex
Ovarian transposition < 45 years of age before RT

Adjuvant radiation therapy (locoregional recurrence decreases): Indications are any one of the following:
- Positive LN
- Parametrial infiltration
- Positive surgical margin
- Any two of the following: Sedlis criteria
  - Large tumor size ≥ 4 cm
  - Deep stromal invasion
  - Positive LVSI

Special Roles of RT:
- Adjuvant hysterectomy after RT (e.g., uterine fibroid limiting the role of Brachy)
- NACT followed by RT
- Intraoperative RT (IORT)—at-risk tumor bed/unresectable-isolated area
- Hemostatic RT (400 cGy-3 days and then change to conventional method/20 Gy in 5#)
- Interstitial implants
- Pregnancy with Ca cervix as adjuvant RT because pregnancy usually causes delay in treatment and, hence, RT added after Sx
- Palliative RT for recurrence

Contd...

Contd...

Conventional RT in Ca Cervix:
- EBRT:
  1.8–2.0 Gy # per day × 5 days = 200 cGy × 5 = 1,000 cGy per week
  5 weeks = 5000 cGy = 50 Gy in 25# to 28#
- CCRT: Cisplatin 50 mg/week 4#–5# (decrease in recurrence by 50%)
- ICRT/brachytherapy:
  - 5.5 to 6 Gy × 5 #
  - 7 Gy × 3 # (usually given)

Interstitial brachytherapy applicators indications:
- Bulky barrel-shaped disease
- Narrow/obliterated vagina
- Obliterated fornices
- Stenotic/obliterated endocervical canal
- Recurrent disease

- **Clinical applications of RT in endometrial cancer:**

Role of RT in Ca endometrium after the surgicopathological staging:
- Stage I A G1 and G2: Observation or VBT if risk factors positive
- Stage I A G3: VBT
- Stage I B G1 and G2: VBT
- Stage I B G3: VBT ± EBRT ± Systemic chemotherapy
- Stage II G1 and G2: VBT ± EBRT
- Stage II G3: EBRT± VBT ± Systemic chemotherapy
- Stage III A–IV A: EBRT ± VBT ± systemic chemotherapy/systemic therapy ± VBT
- Stage IV B: Systemic therapy ± EBRT ± VBT

RT mode are:
- Adjuvant RT (tumor directed RT): Not later than 12 weeks after Sx
- EBRT
- Brachytherapy
- Extended field radiation

Risk factors: Age > 60 years, myometrial invasion > 50% and LVSI positive, etc.

Role of RT in other uterine malignancies:
- Leiomyosarcoma: No benefit
- Endometrial stromal sarcoma: No benefit
- Undifferentiated uterine sarcoma: ± may decrease recurrences without improvement in OS
- Carcinosarcomas: ± may decrease recurrences without improvement in OS

- **Clinical applications of RT in vulval cancer:**

Definitive radiotherapy: Advanced disease or poor surgical candidates
Adjuvant therapy: Tumor-directed EBRT:
- Close/positive margin
- LVSI positive
- >5 mm depth of invasion
- Groin involvement (LN with >2 micro-mets or 1 macro-mets or extracapsular spread) Stage III
- Single SLN positive (≤2 mm mets)

Contd...

Contd...

Primary radiation therapy:
- Advanced disease who otherwise would require pelvic exenteration
- Periclitoral or clitoral lesions in young/middle-aged patients
- Alternative to groin LN dissections palliative radiation therapy: Brachytherapy in special cases
- Adjuvant RT: 45–50.4 Gy in 25–28#
- Primary unresectable disease: 59.4–64.8 Gy in 33–36#
- Chemoradiation: Cisplatin/fluorouracil/mitomycin

- **Use of radiation therapy in other cases in gynecological oncology:**

  - *Ca ovary:* Intraperitoneal radiocolloids and whole abdominal radiation:
    - High morbidity and not used now-a-days
    - Renewed interest in early-staged non-serous types and recurrence
  - *Stage IV GTN (cerebral mets):* 3,000 cGy in 10#
  - *Vaginal cancer:* EBRT + ICRT/interstitial brachytherapy
  - *Special cases:* Paget's disease of vulva and malignant pelvic schwannoma

Surgical Anatomy and Surgical Principles in Gynecological Oncology

1. Gonadal primordia are of what embryological developmental layer?

  a. Ectoderm
  b. Mesoderm
  c. Endoderm
  d. Trophectoderm

2. Primitive germ cells originate from the:

  a. Epiblast
  b. Endoderm
  c. Mesoderm
  d. Ectoderm

3. SRY gene is located in the:

  a. Yp11
  b. Yp12
  c. Yq11
  d. Yq12

4. SRY gene and SOX9 act by:

  a. Tubules from mesonephric ducts penetrate gonadal ridge through FGF9
  b. Stimulates differentiation of sertoli cells and leydig cells by SF1
  c. Elevates the concentration of the antimüllerian hormone (AMH)
  d. All of the above

5. WNT4, RSPO1, and DAX1 act by:

  a. Inhibiting SOX9
  b. Differentiation of the primitive ovary
  c. Estrogen also stimulates the paramesonephric ducts
  d. All of the above

6. Meiosis I of the primary oocyte is arrested until ovulation in what stage of cell division?

  a. Leptotene
  b. Zygotene
  c. Pachytene
  d. Diplotene

7. Number of oogonia at the time of puberty:

  a. 300,000–500,000
  b. 30,000–50,000
  c. 3,000–5,000
  d. 300–400

8. The superficial fatty subcutaneous layer of vulva is known as:

  a. Camper fascia
  b. Scarpa fascia
  c. Colles fascia
  d. None of the above

9. Origin of pudendal nerve is from:

a. S1–S2
b. S2–S3
c. S3–S4
d. S2–S4

10. All are branches of pudendal artery, *except*:

a. Clitoral artery
b. Perineal artery
c. Inferior hemorrhoidal artery
d. Vaginal artery

11. Nerve supply to levator ani:

a. Anterior branch of the ventral ramus S3–S4
b. Anterior branch of the ventral ramus S2–S4
c. Anterior branch of the ventral ramus S2–S3
d. Posterior branch of the ventral ramus S2–S3

12. Origin of genitofemoral nerve is:

a. L1 and L2
b. L2 and L3
c. L1–L3
d. None of the above

13. Which of the following is not a part of the levator ani muscle complex?

a. Puborectalis
b. Pubococcygeal muscle
c. Iliococcygeal muscle
d. Coccygeal muscle

14. The term parametrium refers to:

a. Cardinal ligament attached to uterus and uterosacral ligament
b. Uterosacral ligament attached to uterus
c. Cardinal ligament portion attached to vagina
d. Broad ligament attached to uterus

15. Frankenhauser ganglion of the inferior hypogastric plexus (pelvic plexus) is:

a. Vesical plexus
b. Uterovaginal plexus
c. Middle rectal plexus
d. Inferior rectal plexus

16. Branches of the anterior division of the internal iliac artery include all, *except*:

a. Obturator artery
b. Superior vesical artery
c. Superior gluteal artery
d. Middle rectal artery

17. Branches of the anterior division of the internal iliac artery include all, *except*:

a. Uterine artery
b. Internal pudendal artery
c. Inferior vesical artery
d. Iliolumbar artery

18. Branches of the anterior division of the internal iliac artery include all, *except*:

a. Superior vesical artery
b. Inferior vesical artery
c. Middle rectal artery
d. Lateral sacral artery

19. Branches of the posterior division of the internal iliac artery include all, *except*:

a. Superior gluteal artery
b. Lateral sacral artery
c. Iliolumbar artery
d. Vaginal artery (inferior vesical)

20. Lymphatic drainage of the anterior two-thirds vagina is primarily to:

a. External iliac nodes
b. Internal iliac nodes
c. Inguinal nodes
d. None of the above

21. Lymphatic drainage of the lower one-third vagina is primarily to:

a. External iliac nodes
b. Internal iliac nodes
c. Inguinal nodes
d. None of the above

22. What is the dermatone at umbilicus?

a. T10
b. T11
c. T12
d. None of the above

23. "Fibers of Luschka" connect vagina to:

a. Levator ani
b. Urethra
c. Perineal body
d. Pouch of Douglas

24. Amount of smooth muscle presents in the cervix:

a. 10%
b. 20%
c. 30%
d. 80%

25. Lymphatics from the proximal part of vagina are:

a. External iliac lymph nodes
b. Internal iliac lymph nodes
c. Inguinal lymph nodes
d. None of the above

26. The term parametrium refers to:

a. Uterosacral ligament only
b. Cardinal ligament only
c. Both uterosacral ligament and cardinal ligament
d. Uterosacral ligament, cardinal ligament, and paracolpium (vaginal cardinal ligament)

27. Pelvic diaphragm is composed of all the following muscles, *except*:

a. Iliococcygeus
b. Transverse perinei
c. Puborectalis
d. Pubococcygeus

28. Perception of excessive pain on gentle touch is known as:

a. Myofascial pain
b. Allodynia
c. Neuropathic pain
d. Hyperalgesia

29. Present perception of pain theory is known as:

a. Gate control theory
b. Neuromatrix theory
c. Neuroplasticity theory
d. Cartesian theory

30. **Ovarian nerve supply is:**
   a. Parasympathetic only
   b. Sympathetic only
   c. Both motor and sensory parasympathetic and sympathetic nerves
   d. Autonomic only

31. **Which of the following contributes to the "white line"?**
   a. Fascia of obturator internus muscle
   b. Fascia of transversus perineal muscle
   c. Fascia of puborectalis muscle
   d. Fascia of iliopsoas muscle

32. **Inferior epigastric artery is a branch of:**
   a. Internal iliac artery
   b. External iliac artery
   c. Femoral artery
   d. Hypogastric artery

33. **Superficial epigastric artery is a branch of:**
   a. Internal iliac artery
   b. External iliac artery
   c. Hypogastric artery
   d. Femoral artery

34. **All are true regarding pudendal nerve and artery, *except*:**
   a. Perineal branch of the pudendal artery is the largest of the three branches
   b. Three branches are namely: clitoral, perineal, and inferior hemorrhoidal
   c. Arises from the sacral plexus
   d. Pudendal nerve provides only sensory innervation to the perineum

35. **Which of the following is not a part of the vulva?**
   a. Mons
   b. Labia majora and minora
   c. Clitoris
   d. Vestibule
   e. Anus

36. **Components of vagina include:**
   a. Anterior and posterior columns
   b. Carina of urethra
   c. Vaginal sulci and fornices
   d. All of the above

37. **According to Piver's classification of hysterectomy; modified radical hysterectomy is classified as:**
   a. Type I
   b. Type II
   c. Type III
   d. Type IV

38. **According to Querleu and Morrow's classification of hysterectomy: transection of the paracervix at the ureter with removal of lateral paracervical lymph nodes is classified as:**
   a. Type A
   b. Type B1
   c. Type B2
   d. Type C1

39. According to Querleu and Morrow's classification of hysterectomy: transection of the paracervix at the junction with the internal iliac vascular system along with preservation of autonomic nerves is classified as:

a. Type C1
b. Type C2
c. Type B2
d. Type D1

40. Lymph node dissection at the level of inframesenteric aortic artery is defined as:

a. Level 1
b. Level 2
c. Level 3
d. Level 4

41. Lymph node dissection at the level of infrarenal vein is defined as:

a. Level 1
b. Level 2
c. Level 3
d. Level 4

42. The lateral boundary of Okabayashi's space is formed by:

a. Uterine artery
b. Ureter
c. Iliac vessels
d. Rectum

43. What is the content of the Okabayashi's (medial pararectal space) space:

a. Inferior hypogastric plexus
b. Nodes
c. Ureter
d. None of the above

44. True about Latzko space are all, *except*:

a. Lateral boundary by iliac vessels
b. Also known as lateral pararectal space
c. Medial boundary by ureter
d. Also known as medial pararectal space

45. True about Yabuki's space are all, *except*:

a. Lined by peritoneal epithelial cells
b. Lined by cervicovesical fascia
c. Contains parasympathetic nerves innervating bladder
d. known as third space in pelvis

46. The most important means to prevent ureteral injury is:

a. Surgical knowledge of the location and anatomy of the ureter
b. Preoperative intravenous pyelogram
c. Administration of intravenous indigo carmine during surgery
d. Prophylactic ureteral stent placement

47. The most common gynecologic surgical procedure causing ureteral damage is:

a. Total vaginal hysterectomy
b. Bladder neck dissection

    c. Total abdominal hysterectomy
    d. Total laparoscopic hysterectomy

48. **The most common site of ureteral injury during pelvic surgery is:**
    a. Intramural portion of ureter
    b. Infundibulopelvic ligament at the pelvic brim
    c. Crossing of ureter and uterine artery at the cardinal ligament
    d. Tunnel of Wertheim

49. **Main advantage of radical surgery over radiation therapy in an operable case of cancer cervix:**
    a. Better survival advantage with surgery
    b. Preservation of ovarian function with surgery
    c. Less complication with surgery
    d. Decreased short-term recurrence

50. **In type II radical hysterectomy; uterine artery is ligated at:**
    a. Crossing of the ureter
    b. Origin of the anterior division of the internal iliac artery
    c. Tunnel of Wertheim
    d. Close to the uterus

51. **In type III radical hysterectomy; uterine artery is ligated at:**
    a. Crossing of the ureter
    b. Origin of the anterior division of the internal iliac artery
    c. Tunnel of Wertheim
    d. Close to the uterus

52. **The most common late complication of radical hysterectomy is:**
    a. Vesicovaginal fistula   b. Lower limb numbness
    c. Bladder dysfunction   d. Leg edema

53. **"Terrible triad" in a case of cancer cervix includes all, *except*:**
    a. Unilateral ureteral obstruction   b. Sciatic nerve pain
    c. Unilateral leg edema   d. Vesicovaginal fistula

54. **According to Reiffenstuhl's concepts of lymphatic drainage of cervix: Radical hysterectomy and pelvic lymphadenectomy do not remove the following group of lymph nodes:**
    a. Gluteal lymph nodes   b. Sacral lymph nodes
    c. Rectal lymph nodes   d. All of the above

55. **Damage to the obturator nerve causes:**
    a. Motor impairment to the adductor muscles of the thigh
    b. Sensory impairment of the medial part of the thigh
    c. Origin is from anterior division of L2, L3, and L4
    d. All of the above

56. **All are true in radical trachelectomy, *except*:**

a. Uterine artery is transected
b. Cervicovaginal artery is transected
c. Cervix is amputated 1 cm distal to the isthmus
d. Tumor free margin of at least 8–10 mm
e. All of the above

57. **Indication of Dargent procedure (radical vaginal hysterectomy and laparoscopic pelvic lymphadenectomy) include all, *except*:**

a. No nodal metastasis
b. No involvement of the endocervical region
c. Stage I A1, Stage I A2, and Stage I B1
d. Only squamous cell carcinoma

58. **What is the rate of successful viable pregnancy above 32 weeks gestation after radical vaginal trachelectomy?**

a. 30% approximately
b. 50% approximately
c. 70% approximately
d. 80% approximately

59. **Which of the following is a relative contraindication to exenteration surgery?**

a. Obesity
b. Mental retardation
c. Renal failure
d. Age > 70 years

60. **Unresectable tumor in pelvic exenteration is suggestive by all, *except*:**

a. Unilateral leg edema
b. Vesicovaginal fistula
c. Sciatic nerve pain
d. Unilateral ureteral obstruction

61. **Use of myocutaneous flap for vaginal reconstruction during pelvic exenteration has the following characteristics, *except*:**

a. Pelvic defect is filled up by it
b. Brings in new blood supply to pelvis
c. Postoperative vaginal obturator is not required
d. Requires less training to perform it

62. **Absolute contraindication to do a rectus abdominis myocutaneous flap is:**

a. Previous radiotherapy
b. Obesity
c. Previous hernia surgery
d. Previous Maylard incision

63. **Success of sigmoid neovagina procedure depends upon incorporating the following artery:**

a. Dorsal clitoral artery
b. Superior hemorrhoidal artery
c. Inferior hemorrhoidal artery
d. Pudendal artery

64. During a gracilis myocutaneous flap procedure; gracilis muscle is usually confused with:

a. Adductor magnus
b. Adductor longus
c. Adductor brevis
d. Sartorius

65. All of the following are considered disadvantages of the traditional vulvectomy, *except*:

a. Wound breakdown
b. Perineal contractions
c. Urinary incontinence
d. Increased risk of recurrence

66. Components of Z-plasty pedicle flap include all, *except*:

a. Flap length of 2 cm and a base of 1 cm
b. Full-thickness skin graft
c. Adequate blood supply
d. Rotation of the flap to the midperineal line
   (the ideal rule is that a 2 cm base should be present for each 1 cm length of the flap)

67. Physiologic characteristics of continent urinary pouch are designed to achieve:

a. 80 cm H_2O pressure and 500 mL volume
b. 40 cm H_2O pressure and 500 mL volume
c. 40 cm H_2O pressure and 1,000 mL volume
d. 80 cm H_2O pressure and 1,000 mL volume
   (to prevent infection, reflux and incontinence)

68. Vaginal reconstruction in pelvic exenteration surgery has the advantage of all, *except*:

a. Psychological benefit
b. Beneficial for wound healing
c. Decreases the chances of fistula
d. Increases chance of pelvic collection

69. True about gracilis myocutaneous graft includes:

a. Main supply to the pedicle is from medial circumflex artery
b. Innervation is from obturator nerve
c. Smaller flap can reduce the chance of flap necrosis
d. Infection can complicate 37% cases
e. All are true

70. Techniques for vaginal reconstruction after pelvic exenteration are:

a. Gracilis myocutaneous flap
b. Omental J-flap with split-thickness skin graft
c. Sigmoid neovagina
d. Rectus abdominis myocutaneous flap
e. All of the above

71. **Boundaries of the femoral triangle include all, *except*:**

a. Medial border of adductor longus (medially)
b. Medial border of sartorius (laterally)
c. Lateral border of adductor longus (medially)
d. Inguinal ligament (base)

72. **How many branches of femoral artery are there in the femoral triangle?**

a. Six
b. Four
c. Two
d. Eight

73. **Greater omentum has got how many layers of the peritoneum?**

a. Two
b. Three
c. Four
d. Single

74. **Criteria for fertility preserving surgery in ovarian cancer patients:**

a. No evidence of dysgenetic gonads
b. Close follow-up is feasible
c. Any unilateral malignant germ cell tumor/sex cord-stromal tumor/ borderline tumor
d. Stage I A invasive epithelial tumor
e. All of the above

75. **True about ligation of the hypogastric artery includes all, *except*:**

a. Pulse pressure distal to the point of ligation is decreased by 77% on the same side of ligation
b. Pulse pressure distal to the point of ligation is decreased by 85% when both sides are ligated
c. Blood flow is decreased by 48% at a point distal to the point of ligation
d. All of the above

76. **Risk factor for burst abdomen or evisceration includes all, *except*:**

a. Wound infection
b. Midline incision
c. Ileus
d. Obesity

77. **In general; the wound infection rate in nonobese patients undergoing surgery:**

a. 4–10%
b. 10–15%
c. 20–25%
d. 25–30%

78. **In general; the wound infection rate in obese patients undergoing surgery:**

a. 4–10%
b. 10–15%
c. 20–25%
d. 25–30%

79. Which is the most common cause of fascial dehiscence?

    a. Suture knot failure   b. Suture breakage
    c. Suture pulling through fascia   d. Wound infection

ANSWERS KEY

1. b	2. a	3. a	4. d	5. d	6. d	7. a
8. a	9. d	10. d	11. a	12. a	13. a	14. a
15. b	16. c	17. d	18. d	19. d	20. b	21. c
22. a	23. a	24. a	25. b	26. c	27. b	28. b
29. b	30. c	31. a	32. b	33. d	34. d	35. e
36. d	37. b	38. c	39. a	40. c	41. d	42. b
43. a	44. d	45. d	46. a	47. c	48. c	49. b
50. a	51. b	52. c	53. d	54. d	55. d	56. e
57. d	58. d	59. d	60. b	61. d	62. d	63. b
64. d	65. d	66. a	67. a	68. d	69. e	70. e
71. c	72. a	73. c	74. d	75. d	76. d	77. a
78. d	79. c					

NOTES: SURGICAL ANATOMY AND SURGICAL PRINCIPLES

- Increased risk of portsite metastasis occurs in presence of ascites or peritoneal disease.
- Intraoperative rupture of malignant ovarian masses is a cause of poor prognosis compared to no rupture or spill in early-stage ovarian cancer. Because of the risk of peritoneal dissemination; it is recommended that definitive surgery should be performed within 1 week in ruptured stage I cases.
- Carbon dioxide (CO_2) peritoneum and intra-abdominal pressure ≥ 12 mm Hg are risk factors of malignant dissemination according to some studies.
- In radical trachelectomy; the uterus is divided 5 mm below the isthmus. Dargent approach is the gold standard of radical trachelectomy.

- Middle rectal artery is an important landmark separating the neural part from the vascular part of the paracervix. This is an important concept in the nerve-sparing radical hysterectomy (type C1).
- LAP2 in endometrial cancer showed comparable recurrence (11.4% in laparoscopy and 10.2% in laparotomy) and over-all 5 year survival was identical in both the arms (89.8%).
- Laparoscopic Approach to Cervical Cancer (LACC) Trial (2019): Minimally invasive versus abdominal radical hysterectomy in cervical cancer. Stage IA1 (lymphovascular invasion), IA2, or IB1 cervical cancer and a histologic subtype of squamous-cell carcinoma, adenocarcinoma, or adenosquamous carcinoma were included in this trial. In this trial, minimally invasive radical hysterectomy was associated with lower rates of disease-free survival and overall survival than open abdominal radical hysterectomy among women with early-stage cervical cancer.
- Advantages of robotic surgery in gynecologic oncology:
  - There is increased dexterity, improved vision, and faster learning curve.
  - Reduced complication rate, pain, bleeding, and length of hospital stay compared to open surgery.
  - There is reduced conversion rate compared to laparoscopy.
  - Lymph node yield is comparable to laparoscopy and increased when compared to laparotomy.
- Disadvantages of robotic surgery in gynecologic oncology:
  - Short-term and long-term oncological outcome are evolving.
  - Increased operating time compared to the open surgery.
  - Lack of haptics.
  - Cost of installation and maintenance is high.
- HAL = Hand-assisted laparoscopy.
- NOTES = Natural orifice transluminal endoscopic surgery.
- *Pelvic vasculature*: Internal iliac artery
  - Anterior branches (Ist medial branch is the uterine artery, 1st lateral branch is obturator artery, internal pudendal artery, superior vesical artery, inferior vesical or vaginal artery, middle rectal artery)
  - Posterior branches (Superior gluteal artery, Iliolumbar artery and Lateral sacral artery)
- Lymphatic drainage of vulva:
  - Lymphatics from the vulva and the distal third of the vagina drain to the superficial inguinal lymph nodes (T-shaped distribution consisting of 15-20 numbers and is being divided into four quadrants by the saphenous opening as the center of the quadrant) and from here they enter the deep inguinal nodes (3-4 nos) situated in the femoral canal. Cloquet node is the superior most deep femoral lymph nodes. Lymphatics from the upper third of vulva, within 2 cm from the mid-line and clitoris drain to bilateral inguinal lymph nodes while lymphatics from the lower third of the vulva drain to unilateral inguinal lymph nodes.

- *Boundaries of the femoral triangle*: Base by the inguinal ligament, laterally by the medial border of the Sartorius muscle and medially by the lateral border of the Adductor longus.
- Lymphatic drainage from the cervix follows the uterine arteries and cardinal ligaments to the pelvic nodes that include the external iliac, internal iliac (hypogastric), and obturator nodes. From these pelvic lymph nodes, the drainage proceeds superiorly through the common iliac and presacral lymph nodes and then up to the para-aortic lymph nodes.
- Lymphatic drainage from the uterine corpus and the ovaries goes along the routes of the uterine arteries in the broad ligaments to the pelvic lymph nodes, along the round ligaments to the inguinal lymph nodes and along the ovarian lymphatics in the infundibulopelvic ligaments directly up to the para-aortic lymph nodes.
- There are six groups of retroperitoneal para-aortic lymph nodes. They are: paracaval, retrocaval, interaortocaval, preaortic, para-aortic, and retroaortic groups of lymph nodes. The preaortic drains the abdominal part of the gastrointestinal tract down to the midrectum, whereas the retrocaval and the retroaortic groups have no special areas of drainage. The precaval, interaortocaval, and para-aortic lymph nodes receive lymphatic drainage from the iliac nodes, ovaries, and other pelvic viscera and these groups are essentially sampled in case of gynecologic malignancy. However, para-aortic lymph nodes dissection should address all the six groups of lymph nodes of the para-aortic regions. Low para-aortic lymph node dissection is carried up to the origin of the inferior mesenteric artery. The upper boundary of full PALND is up to the origin of the renal veins. The approach to PALND is either by Transperitoneal approach or by Kocher's maneuver.
- The boundaries of pelvic lymph node basin: *Laterally* by genito-femoral nerve, *Medially* by the anterior branch of the internal iliac artery and subsequently by its obliterated extension, *Posteriorly* by the obturator nerve and *Inferiorly* by the circumflex-iliac vein.
- Anatomical spaces in gynecological oncology surgery:
  - Space of Retzius (pre-vesical)
  - Space of Bogros (retro-inguinal)
  - Para-vesical space
  - Para-rectal space
  - Vesico-vaginal space
  - Recto-vaginal space
  - Obturator space
  - Pre-sacral space
  - Yabuki's space (Fourth space)
  - Okabayashi space (Medial para-rectal space)
  - Latzko space (Lateral para-rectal space)
- There are various types of lymphadenectomies namely systemic lymphadenectomy, debulking lymphadenectomy, lymph node dissection, diagnostic lymphadenectomy, sentinel lymph node biopsy, etc.

- The origin of the inferior mesenteric artery is about 4–5 cm above the aortic bifurcation.
- The right and the left ovarian arteries originate from the respective sides of the aorta about 3–4 cm above the bifurcation of the aorta.
- The right ovarian vein inserts into the right side of the inferior vena cava (IVC) about 1–2 cm below the insertion of the left renal vein.
- There are four pairs of lumbar arteries and veins that arise from the posterior surfaces of the aorta and IVC, respectively. There is a pair of "fellows vein" in the front of IVC about 3 cm from the bifurcation.
- Line of Toldt in the lateral part of the paracolic gutters are used for the mobilization required for the para-aortic lymph node dissection.
- Approaches to para-aortic lymphadenectomy include: transperitoneal, extraperitoneal, open, or laparoscopic/robotic.
- Lymphadenectomy in Ovarian Neoplasm (LION) Study result (2017): Systematic pelvic and para-aortic lymphadenectomy (LNE) in patients with advanced ovarian cancer (AOC) with both intra-abdominal complete resection and clinically negative LN neither improve overall nor progression-free survival despite detecting (and removing) subclinical retroperitoneal lymph node metastases in 56% of the patients. Our data indicate that systematic LNE of clinical negative LN in patients with AOC and complete resection should be omitted to reduce postoperative morbidity and mortality.
- *Exploratory laparotomy*: When the diagnosis is not well-established before surgery and may proceed according to the intra-operative findings.
- *Primary cytoreductive surgery*: It is the initial surgery (usually a laparotomy) to establish a diagnosis, stage and attempt to remove maximal tumor burden to microscopic level before initiation of the first-line chemotherapy. Complete cytoreduction means cytoreduction of all tumors independent of preoperative tumor load to microscopic residual disease at the time of completion of surgery with no gross residual tumors left (R0 resection). Macroscopic disease up to 1 cm in diameter after primary surgery (optimal cytoreduction or R 1 resection). Primary cytoreduction resulting in macroscopic disease larger than 1 cm in size at the end of surgery (sub-optimal cytoreduction or R 2 resection).
- *Secondary cytoreductive surgery*: Usually done in oligometastatic recurrent disease in post-primary debulking and/or chemotherapy. It is done in platinum sensitive disease and with disease free interval of about two years.

Enhanced Recovery after Surgery (ERAS)

Preoperative Care

- Optimized medical/health condition
- Informed decision and patient education

- Preoperative health and risk assessment
- Optimized hydration and nutrition
- Reduced starvation
- Patient information and expectation managed
- Discharge planning
- No or reduced bowel preparation.

Intraoperative

- MIS or transverse incision
- No nasogastric tube
- Use of local anesthetic with sedation
- Epidural management
- Optimized fluid management.

Postoperative

- Planned mobilization
- Rapid hydration and nourishment
- Appropriate IV therapy
- No wound drains
- No nasogastric tube
- Catheters removed early
- Regular oral analgesics
- Avoidance of opiate analgesics.

Discharge

- Early discharge date with full information and ongoing support
- Allied health support
- Personal follow-up from clinical team.

Gynecological cancers	Type of staging
GTN	FIGO clinical staging WHO risk stratification staging
Vulva	Surgicopathological staging
Vagina	Clinical staging
Cervix	Surgicopathological and radiological staging
Uterine sarcoma	Surgicopathological staging
Endometrial	Surgicopathological staging
Ovary, fallopian tube, and primary peritoneal	Surgicopathological staging

(FIGO: International Federation of Gynecology and Obstetrics staging system; GTN: gestational trophoblastic neoplasia; WHO: World Health Organization)

- Peritoneal Cancer Index is an intra-operative integration of both peritoneal implant size and distribution of nodules on the peritoneal surface. Abdomen is divided in to 13 abdomino-pelvic regions namely; central, right upper, epigastrium, left upper, left flank, left lower, pelvis, right lower, right flank, upper jejunum, lower jejunum, upper ileum and lower ileum. Lesion size score (LS-0 no tumor seen, LS-1 tumor up to 0.5 cm, LS-2 tumor up to 5.0 cm and LS-3 tumor > 5.0 cm or confluence)
- Completeness of cytoreduction score after surgery (CC Score): CC-0 (No disease), CC-1 (Present to 0.25 cm), CC-2 (0.25 cm to 2.5 cm) and CC-3 (>2.5 cm)

Pathology in Gynecological Oncology

1. **Psammoma bodies along with large cytoplasmic vacuoles imply:**
   a. Serous carcinoma
   b. Mucinous carcinoma
   c. Squamous carcinoma
   d. Normal endometrial cells

2. **Hybrid capture II (HC2) test for human papillomavirus (HPV) deoxyribonucleic acid (DNA) has got increased sensitivity and decreased specificity due to:**
   a. Cross-reactivity
   b. Leak of chemiluminescent signal from contiguous samples
   c. Very high viral loads of low-risk HPV
   d. All of the above

3. **True about neuroendocrine carcinoma of cervix includes all, *except*:**
   a. Aggressive variety
   b. Deeply invasive variety
   c. Non-HPV related
   d. p16 positive

4. **True about endocervical adenocarcinoma includes all, *except*:**
   a. ER negative and PR negative
   b. Vimentin negative
   c. Dimorphic patterns of endometrial cells
   d. p16 negative

5. **Most common malignant glandular lesion in the vagina is:**
   a. Endometrial adenocarcinoma
   b. Mucinous adenocarcinoma
   c. Mesonephric adenocarcinoma
   d. Clear cell adenocarcinoma

6. **The type of cervical carcinoma which is not related to HPV is:**
   a. Adenoma malignum
   b. Villoglandular carcinoma
   c. Mesonephric carcinoma
   d. Neuroendocrine carcinoma

7. **Most common site of vaginal melanoma is:**
   a. Anterior wall of the lower one-third vagina
   b. Anterior wall of the upper one-third vagina
   c. Posterior wall of lower one-third vagina
   d. Posterior wall of upper one-third vagina

8. Most common type of HPV related to vulval intraepithelial neoplasia 2 (VIN 2) and VIN 3 is:

a. HPV 16
b. HPV 18
c. HPV 31
d. HPV 33

9. Premalignant potential of atypical complex endometrial hyperplasia is:

a. 5%
b. 10%
c. 20%
d. 30%

10. Endometrial cancer includes all, *except* (differentiates from endocervical cancers):

a. ER positive and PR positive
b. Vimentin positive
c. p16 negative
d. HPV positive

11. Tamoxifen-related endometrial cancer is:

a. Endometrial adenocarcinoma
b. Serous carcinoma
c. Clear cell carcinoma
d. Mucinous adenocarcinoma

(Tamoxifen is also associated with ovarian cysts, endometrial polyps and uterine sarcoma. Some studies implicate clear cell endometrial carcinoma also from Tamoxifen use but till now not mentioned in the standard books. However, clear cell carcinoma of cervix is associated with DES exposure in utero)

12. Hobnail or tombstone appearance is characteristics of:

a. Endometrioid adenocarcinoma
b. Serous carcinoma
c. Clear cell carcinoma
d. Mucinous adenocarcinoma

13. International Federation of Gynecology and Obstetrics (FIGO) grade 3 endometrial carcinoma displays solid epithelial growth of:

a. >5%
b. 6–50%
c. >50%
d. >60%

14. Mitotic figures per 10 high power fields in smooth muscle tumor of uncertain malignant potential (STUMP) include:

a. 5 to 10
b. < 5
c. > 10
d. None of the above

15. Clinically benign condition includes:

a. Atypical leiomyoma
b. Metastasizing leiomyoma
c. Diffuse leiomyomatosis
d. All of the above

(NB: Intravenous leiomyomatosis and disseminated peritoneal leiomyomatosis are alsobenign conditions)

16. Characteristics of endometrial stromal nodule include all, *except*:

a. Benign
b. No LVSI
c. No myometrial invasion
d. Myometrial infiltration present

17. **Prior pelvic irradiation has been associated with:**

  a. Adenosarcoma
  b. Atypical polypoidal adenomyoma
  c. Endometrial stromal sarcoma
  d. Carcinosarcoma

18. **Borderline ovarian tumors are characterized by all, *except*:**

  a. Mean age of 45 years at diagnosis
  b. About 15% of ovarian neoplasms
  c. Lymph node involvement
  d. Absence of endosalpingiosis

19. **Borderline ovarian tumors are may include:**

  a. Implants   b. Micropapillary pattern
  c. Stromal microinvasion   d. Lymph nodal involvement
  e. All of the above

20. **Which is the most common malignant ovarian tumor associated with BRCA mutations?**

  a. High grade serous tumor
  b. Primary peritoneal carcinoma
  c. Primary fallopian tube carcinoma
  d. Low grade serous carcinoma

21. **Definition of stromal microinvasion found in borderline ovarian tumor is:**

  a. 2 mm in linear extent or 4 mm^2 area
  b. 3 mm in linear extent or 6 mm^2 area
  c. 4 mm in linear extent or 8 mm^2 area
  d. 5 mm in linear extent or 10 mm^2 area

22. **Which amongst the following type of mucinous ovarian tumor is associated with endometriosis?**

  a. Mucinous tumor with pseudomyxoma peritonei
  b. Mucinous tumor of intestinal type
  c. Mullerian mucinous borderline tumor
  d. Benign mucinous tumor

23. **What percentage of endometrioid ovarian carcinoma is associated with endometriosis?**

  a. 10%   b. 20%
  c. 30%   d. 40%

(Correct answer noted is as per 6th Edition of Berek and Hacker's Gynecologic Oncology page no-192). (But 6th Edition Principles and Practice of Gynecologic Oncology page no 802: 15% to 20%)

24. **What percentage of endometrioid ovarian carcinoma is associated with primary endometrioid endometrial carcinoma?**
a. 5% to 10%
b. 14% to 20%
c. 25% to 30%
d. 2% to 5%

25. **True about clear cell ovarian carcinoma is all, *except*:**
a. Increase prevalence in Japan
b. 2/3rd associated with nulliparity
c. 50% are associated with endometriosis
d. ARIDIA mutations not seen in endometriosis associated types

26. **Clear cell ovarian carcinoma includes all, *except*:**
a. Hobnail cells
b. Paraneoplastic syndrome
c. Pelvic venous thrombosis
d. Usually bilateral

27. **Clear cell carcinoma includes all, *except*:**
a. Not graded
b. Unilateral
c. Infertility
d. Young age at presentation

28. **Endometriosis-associated ovarian tumor includes all, *except*:**
a. Pseudomyxoma peritonei
b. Endometrioid ovarian carcinoma
c. Clear cell ovarian carcinoma
d. ARIDIA mutations

29. **True about Walthard bodies includes:**
a. Transitional type epithelial inclusions
b. Subserosal location
c. Benign
d. All of the above

30. **Brenner ovarian tumor includes all, *except*:**
a. Solid with small cystic spaces
b. Associated with mucinous cystic spaces
c. Malignant transitional cells associated with benign or atypical proliferating transitional elements
d. Malignant transitional cells without benign or atypical proliferating transitional elements
(Malignant transitional cells without benign or atypical proliferating transitional elements are designated as Transitional cell carcinoma and not as Brenner's)

31. **Most common sex-cord stromal tumor of ovary is:**
a. Adult granulosa cell tumor
b. Juvenile granulosa cell tumor
c. Sertoli–Leydig cell tumor
d. Fibroma-thecoma

32. **Call–Exner bodies are characteristic of:**

a. Adult granulosa cell tumor
b. Yolk-sac tumor
c. Dysgerminoma
d. Sertoli–Leydig cell tumor

33. **Schiller–Duval bodies are characteristic of:**

a. Adult granulosa cell tumor
b. Yolk-sac tumor
c. Dysgerminoma
d. Sertoli–Leydig cell tumor

34. **True about juvenile granulosa cell tumor includes all, *except*:**

a. Isosexual pseudoprecocity
b. Mostly below 30 years
c. Unilateral and early stage
d. 90% develop recurrences

35. **Sertoli–Leydig cell tumor includes all, *except*:**

a. 50% shows no endocrinologic manifestations
b. 33% shows virilization
c. Unilateral and low stage
d. 50% shows extra-ovarian spread at diagnosis

36. **Peutz–Jeghers syndrome is associated with:**

a. Sex-cord tumor with annular tubules
b. Gynandroblastoma
c. Juvenile granulosa cell tumor
d. Fibroma-thecoma

37. **Reinke crystals are characteristics of:**

a. Steroid cell tumor
b. Leydig cell tumor
c. Stromal luteomas
d. Fibroma-thecoma

38. **Poor prognosis in immature teratoma includes all, *except*:**

a. Mature glial implants in peritoneum (mature gliomatosis peritonei)
b. Greater immature neuroepithelium
c. Grade of the lesion
d. Stage of the lesion

39. **Most frequent type of malignant transformation of a mature teratoma is:**

a. Adenocarcinomas
b. Sarcomas
c. Carcinoids
d. Squamous cell carcinomas

40. **Dysgerminomas include all, *except*:**

a. Expresses PLAP, CD 117, LDH
b. Majority with late diagnosis
c. Most common in gonadal dysgenesis
d. Most common bilateral germ cell tumor

41. **Yolk sac tumor includes all, *except*:**

   a. Expresses AFP, cytokeratin, SALL 4, and glypican
   b. Unilateral and solid   c. Mean age of 20 years
   d. Schiller-Duval bodies   e. All of the above

42. **Paraneoplastic hypercalcemia is associated with:**

   a. Yolk sac tumor   b. Sertoli–Leydig cell tumor
   c. Steroid cell tumor   d. Small cell carcinoma

43. **Most common source of metastatic ovarian carcinoma is:**

   a. Colon   b. Breast
   c. Stomach   d. Pancreas

44. **Classical Krukenberg's (metastatic signet ring) carcinoma includes all, *except*:**

   a. Bilateral disease   b. Surface nodules
   c. Diameter < 10 cm   d. Most commonly from stomach
   e. Less lymphatic involvement

45. **p57 is present in:**

   a. Complete hydatidiform mole
   b. Partial hydatidiform mole
   c. Both a and b
   d. None of the above

46. **True about partial hydatidiform mole includes all, *except*:**

   a. 69 XXY and 69 XYY
   b. Embryonic tissue present
   c. Scalloping of chorionic villi present
   d. 46 XX and 46 XY

47. **What percentage of simple endometrial hyperplasia without atypia will progress to endometrial cancer?**

   a. 1%   b. 3%
   c. 8%   d. 29%

48. **What percentage of complex endometrial hyperplasia without atypia will progress to endometrial cancer?**

   a. 1%   b. 3%
   c. 8%   d. 29%

49. **What percentage of simple atypical hyperplasia will progress to endometrial cancer?**

   a. 1%   b. 3%
   c. 8%   d. 29%

50. **What percentage of complex atypical hyperplasia will progress to endometrial cancer?**

a. 1%

b. 3%

c. 8%

d. 29%

51. **What percentage of endometrial intraepithelial neoplasia will progress to endometrial cancer within 1 year follow-up?**

a. 3%

b. 8%

c. 29%

d. 40%

ANSWERS KEY

1. a	2. d	3. c	4. d	5. d	6. c	7. a
8. a	9. d	10. d	11. d	12. c	13. c	14. a
15. d	16. d	17. d	18. d	19. e	20. a	21. d
22. c	23. d	24. b	25. d	26. d	27. d	28. a
29. d	30. d	31. a	32. a	33. b	34. d	35. d
36. a	37. b	38. a	39. d	40. b	41. e	42. d
43. a	44. e	45. b	46. d	47. a	48. b	49. c
50. d	51. d					

NOTES: ONCOPATHOLOGY

- Immunohistochemistry:

CA Ovary	CK7 +ve, ER +ve, WT +ve, PAX8 +ve, Mesothelin CA125 +ve CK20 Negative
CA Endometrium	ER +ve, PR +ve, Vimentin +ve p16 negative
CA Endocervix	p16 +ve, ER & PR Negative, Vimentin Negative, HPV +ve
CA Cervix	p16 +ve, ER & PR Negative, Vimentin Negative, HPV +ve
GTN	Beta hCG +ve
Sarcoma	Vimentin +ve, CK7 +ve, Desmin +ve S100 Negative & CK 20 Negative
Colorectal CA	CK 20 +ve, CDX2 +ve & CK 7 Negative
CA Bladder (Transitional CA)	CK20 +ve, CK 5/6 +ve, p63+ve, GATA3 +ve, Urothelin +ve
Melanoma	S100 +ve, HMB45 +ve, Melan-A +ve Pan-cytokeratin Negative

- *Most common vaginal sarcoma*: Embryonal rhabdomyosarcoma
- *Vaginal melanoma*: Second most common vaginal malignancy. Most common location of vaginal melanoma is the anterior wall of the lower third of the vagina.
- *High risk HPV virus are (13 types)*: 16, 18, 31, 33, 35, 39, 45, 51, 52, 56, 58, 59 and 66.
- Histologic grading of endometrioid carcinoma:
  - *FIGO Grade 1*: The tumor exhibits well-formed glands and has 5% or less of solid growth pattern
  - *FIGO Grade 2*: The solid growth pattern occupies 6-50% of the tumor
  - *FIGO Grade 3*: The tumor displays more than 50% solid epithelial growth
- Leiomyosarcoma is the most common sarcoma of uterus. The presence of coagulative tumor cell necrosis, cytologic atypia and large numbers of mitotic figures are indicative of leiomyosarcoma.
- *Low-grade endometrial stromal sarcoma*: Usually seen in the pre-menopausal women and confined to the uterus at the time of diagnosis. It has got infiltrating margin, vascular invasion and more than 10 mitotic figures per 10 high-power fields.
- *Borderline ovarian tumor (Low malignant potential)*: Mean age at presentation is 45 years and it constitutes 15% of ovarian serous neoplasms. 10% of them exhibit foci of significant micropapillary architecture and stromal micro-invasion (linear extent of 5 mm or an area of 10 mm^2. 30% to 40% cases may show extra-ovarian implants (non-invasive, invasive or indeterminate). Lymph node involvement may be there in 20% to 30% cases. Endosalpingiosis is also co-exist with borderline ovarian tumors.
- *Low-grade serous ovarian carcinoma*: It is based upon relatively low mitotic index and lower degree of nuclear atypia. It represents less than 10% of malignant ovarian cancer. Mutations commonly seen in these categories include KRAS and BRAF.
- Clear cell carcinoma of the ovary is the most common epithelial ovarian neoplasm to be associated with vascular thrombotic events (18% to 46% cases) and paraneoplastic hypercalcemia (2% to 10% cases).
- *Adult granulosa cell ovarian tumor*: It is characterized by late recurrences and stage of the disease is the most important prognostic factor. Microfollicular Call-Exner bodies and macro-follicular patterns are present and it is associated with the mutations of FOXL2.
- *Juvenile granulosa cell ovarian tumor*: It is associated with isosexual pseudo-precocity or menstrual irregularities and recurrences are seen in 10% cases.
- *Sertoli-Leydig cell ovarian tumor*: 30% present with virilization and is a low stage tumor (and mostly unilateral). Sex-cord tumor with annular tubules is a rare form of it which is associated with Peutz-Jeghers syndrome.

- *Fibroma-Thecoma*: Benign tumors category. 60% of thecomas present with estrogenic manifestations. Fibromas can be associated with ascites and pleural effusion (Meigs syndrome).
- *Yolk sac ovarian tumor*: Characteristic Schiller-Duval bodies along with raised AFP. It is positive for cytokeratin, glypigan-3 and SALL4.
- Cairo and bishop classification for tumor lysis syndrome

Laboratory TLS	*Clinical TLS*
Abnormality in two or more of the following (Occurring within 3 days before or 7 days after chemotherapy)	Laboratory TLS plus one or more of the following
Uric acid > 8 mg/dL or 25% increase	Increased serum creatinine (1.5 times normal value)
Potassium > 6 mEq/L or 25% increase	Cardiac arrhythmia or Sudden death
Phosphate > 4.5 mg/dL or 25% increase	Seizure
Calcium < 7 mg/dL or 25% increase	

(TLS: tumor lysis syndrome)

- Para-neoplastic syndrome:
  - *Ca ovary*: Subacute cerebellar degeneration (Anti-Yo onconeural Ab) and subacute peripheral neuropathy.
  - *Ca cervix*: Lambert-Eaton myasthenia syndrome.
- *Neutropenic fever*: Neutropenia is defined as an absolute neutrophil count of < 500 cells/mm^2 or an expected to be of this value within the next 48 hours. Fever with neutropenia should be considered as evidence of infection. Further reading about risk stratification of febrile neutropenia as per the index of Multinational Association for Supportive Care in Cancer (MASCC).

Tumor Markers and Imaging in Gynecological Oncology

1. Most limiting factor of a tumor marker is:

a. Lack of sensitivity
b. Lack of specificity
c. Costly
d. Lack of positive predictive value

2. True about CA125 includes all, *except*:

a. CA125 is not specific for ovarian cancer
b. M11 and OC125 antibodies are used for CA125
c. CA125 level in ovarian cysts correlate well with serum levels
d. No mortality benefit of screening with CA125 in ovarian cancer

3. Risk of malignancy index includes:

a. CA125, USG score, and menopausal status
b. CA125, color doppler, and menopausal status
c. CA125, cytology of ascitic fluid, and menopausal status
d. CA125, HE4, and USG score

4. Risk of ovarian malignancy algorithm (ROMA) includes:

a. CA125, USG, and menopausal status
b. CA125, color doppler, and menopausal status
c. CA125, HE4, and osteopontin
d. HE4, CA125, and menopausal status

5. Copenhagen index is based upon:

a. Patient age, HE4, and CA125
b. Patient age, USG, and CA125
c. Patient age, USG, and HE4
d. HE4, CA125, and USG

6. Time series risk of ovarian cancer (ROC) algorithm includes all, *except*:

a. Specificity of 98% and sensitivity of 81%
b. Final result is presented with a ROC of 2%
c. Uses CA125 and TVS in triaging
d. Static but elevated levels of CA125 are considered to be high risk

7. **Malignant markers in International Ovarian Tumor Analysis (IOTA) include all, *except*:**

a. Irregular solid tumor
b. Ascites
c. ≥2 papillary structures
d. Irregular multilocular solid tumor with largest diameter ≥10 cm
   (*Note*: Other features of malignant pattern include strong vascularity of tumor and ≥4papillary structures)

8. **Contrast-enhanced transvaginal ultrasound with microbubbles specifically helps indetection of ovarian cancer by:**

a. Pulsatility index
b. Angiogenesis
c. Fluid morphology within the tumor
d. Enhancement of the tumor borders

9. **Lifetime risk of ovarian cancers in BRCA1 carriers is:**

a. 20%   b. 40%
c. 60%   d. 80%
   (*Note*: It is written as 54% in page no. 471 and as 40% in page no. 452 of sixth edition of Berek andHacker's Gynecologic Oncology)

10. **Lifetime risk of ovarian cancers in BRCA2 mutation carriers is:**

a. 18%   b. 28%
c. 38%   d. 48%
   (*Note*: It is written as 23% in page no. 471, 18% in page no. 452, and as 11% in page no. 470 of sixth edition Berek and Hacker's Gynecologic Oncology)

11. ***MMR* gene mutation carriers have a lifetime risk of ovarian cancer is:**

a. 10–12%   b. 15–20%
c. 20–25%   d. 30–35%

12. **Risk of breast cancer in BRCA1 mutations is:**

a. 65%   b. 55%
c. 45%   d. 35%

13. **Risk of breast cancer in BRCA2 mutations is:**

a. 65%   b. 55%
c. 45%   d. 35%

14. **Risk of ovarian malignancy in Lynch syndrome is:**

a. 6–12%   b. 16–20%
c. 24–28%   d. 4–8%

15. *MMR* gene mutations in Lynch syndrome is:

a. *MSH2, MSH3, MLH1, PMS3 and PMS4*
b. *MSH1, MSH3, MLH1, PMS5 and PMS6*
c. *MSH2, MSH3, MLH1, PMS4 and PMS5*
d. *MSH2, MSH6, MLH1, PMS1 and PMS2*

16. In ovarian malignancy, RMI > 200 includes:

a. Sensitivity 84%
b. Specificity 77%
c. PPV 76% and NPV 85%
d. All of the above

17. CA15–3 is used in monitoring response of treatment in:

a. Ovarian cancer
b. Breast cancer
c. Cervical cancer
d. Endometrial cancer

18. Decreased level of human epididymis protein 4 (HE4) is found in all, *except*:

a. Pregnancy
b. Endometriosis
c. Age
d. Germ cell tumors

19. True about HE4 and CA125 in epithelial ovarian cancer (EOC) includes all, *except*:

a. HE4 is low in benign ovarian disease
b. HE4 is a strong and independent prognostic marker than CA125
c. HE4 rises earlier than CA125 in case of recurrence
d. HE4 is inferior to CA125 in early stage EOC and borderline ovarian tumor

20. More accurate markers of gynecologic malignancy in pediatric age group includes all, *except*:

a. Clinical mass per abdomen
b. Ultrasound diagnosis of mass > 8 cm
c. Precocious puberty
d. AFP, CA125, and β-hCG

21. True about corelation of osteopontin in ovarian cancer includes all, *except*:

a. Histologic type of ovarian cancer
b. Presence of ascites
c. Bulky disease load
d. Recurrence

22. Tumor markers found elevated in adult granulosa cell tumor:

a. Inhibin A
b. Inhibin B
c. Anti-müllerian hormone
d. All of the above

23. Squamous cell carcinoma antigen (SCCA) in cervical cancer includes all, *except*:

a. Varies with the grade of the tumor
b. Response to chemotherapy
c. Risk of recurrence
d. Individualizing treatment

24. Recommended as a screening for endometrial cancer in general population in Western countries is:

a. Annual endometrial thickness measurement by TVS
b. Annual CA125
c. Annual endometrial biopsy
d. None of the above

25. Endometrial sampling is needed in a postmenopausal woman when the endometrial thickness is more than:

a. 4 mm
b. 6 mm
c. 8 mm
d. 10 mm

ANSWERS KEY

1. b	2. c	3. a	4. d	5. a	6. d	7. c
8. b	9. b	10. a	11. a	12. a	13. c	14. a
15. d	16. d	17. b	18. c	19. d	20. d	21. a
22. d	23. d	24. d	25. a			

NOTES: TUMOR MARKERS AND IMAGING IN GYNECOLOGIC ONCOLOGY

Endometrial cancer:	
Ultrasound (USG) [Transvaginal sonography (TVS)]	Detection of myometrial invasion by TVS: Sensitivity of 77–100%, specificity 65–93%, and overall accuracy 60–76%
Computed tomography (CT) scan	Detection of myometrial invasion by CT scan: Sensitivity of 83%, specificity 42–93%, and overall accuracy 58–76%. Overall accuracy of detection of recurrence rate is 92%
Magnetic resonance imaging (MRI)	• Detection of myometrial invasion by MRI: Sensitivity of 70–95% and specificity 80–95% • Detection of cervical stromal invasion by MRI: Sensitivity of 75–80%, specificity 94–96%, and overall accuracy 90–92%

Contd...

Contd...

Positron emission tomography (PET) CT scan	<ul><li>Nodal sensitivity for 10 mm is 93.3%</li><li>Distant metastasis sensitivity of 100% and specificity of 94%, detection of recurrence</li></ul>
Gestational trophoblastic neoplasia:	
USG	<ul><li>Heterogenous cystic spaces, increased vascularity, irregular borders ± asymmetric extension of the mass into myometrium</li><li>Enlarged ovarian theca luteal cysts</li></ul>
CT scan	Locoregional spread and metastasis
PET CT scan	Metastasis and recurrence

Cervical cancer:	
USG	Only important role is the detection of the hydronephrosis
CT scan	<ul><li>More useful for advanced disease</li><li>Has limitations like poor detection of primary small tumors, parametrial invasion, and bladder/bowel mucosal involvement</li><li>Sensitivity, specificity, and negative predictive value (NPV) of CT scan in staging cervical cancer of stage II B or more is 42%, 82%, and 84%, respectively</li></ul>
MRI	<ul><li>Single BEST imaging modality</li><li>Accurately detects tumor size, location, parametrial invasion, adjacent organ involvement, and nodal involvement. It is useful in detecting recurrence, complications, and treatment response</li><li>Overall accuracy, specificity, and NPV of MRI in detecting parametrial involvement is 88–97%, 93%, and 94%, respectively</li><li>If the intact peripheral low signal intensity stromal rim of the cervix is >3 mm (hypotensive rim sign), parametrial invasion can almost be excluded with specificity of 96–99% and NPV of 94–100%</li></ul>
PET CT scan	<ul><li>Detection of lymph nodes and metastasis. Useful in surveillance for detection of recurrence</li><li>SUVmax of the primary cervical cancer is a sensitive biomarker of treatment response, prognosis, recurrence risk, and disease-specific survival</li></ul>
Ovarian cancer:	
USG	<ul><li>Detection and characterization of the adnexal mass: solid components, septation, vascularity, papillary structures, ascites, liver metastasis, etc.</li><li>Usually is combined with tumor markers for scoring systems</li></ul>
CT scan	<ul><li>Sensitivity, specificity, and accuracy of distinguishing benign from malignant mass are 89%, 96–99%, and 92–94%, respectively</li><li>Useful in detecting abdominal involvement like peritoneal implants, omental thickening/caking, mesenteric metastasis, lymph nodal involvement, and liver/spleen involvement</li><li>Staging accuracy of CT scan is 70–90%</li><li>BEST imaging modality in ovarian tumor</li></ul>
PET CT scan	Detection of recurrence

- Advantages of CT scan include ready availability, short image acquisition times, large field of view, high spatial resolution, and rapid 3-D reconstructions. Disadvantages include ionizing radiation, image quality loss in case of metallic implants, and morbidity associated with iodinated contrast agents.
- Advantages of MRI include superior soft-tissue contrast, absence of ionizing radiation, multiplanar capability, patient allergic to iodine, or having renal impairment. Disadvantage of MRI includes longer acquisition time and claustrophobia. MRI is contraindicated in patients with pacemakers, cochlear implants, certain vascular clips, metallic objects in eye, and neural simulators.
- Fluorodeoxyglucose (FDG)-PET CT scan gives a biochemical as well as structural changes but spatial resolution or soft tissue contrast is low when compared to other imaging modalities.
- RMI (Jacob et al., 1990) is an algorithm based on scores derived from ultrasound variables, menopausal status, and serum CA-125 level. RMI I, II, III, and IV have been established and generally accepted by clinicians to distinguish malignant ovarian tumors from benign ones. Ultrasound characters include-multilocular cystic lesion, solid areas, bilateral lesions, ascites, intra-abdominal metastases.

Variants	Ultrasound score (U)	Menopausal score (M)	Tumor size (S) cm
RMI I = U × M × CA-125 Cut off -200	U = 0 (0 parameter) U = 1 (1 parameter) U = 3 (≥2 parameters)	M = 1(premenopausal) M = 3(postmenopausal)	Not applicable
RMI II = U × M × CA-125 Cut off -200	U = 1 (0/1 parameter) U = 4 (≥2 parameters)	M = 1(premenopausal) M = 4(postmenopausal)	Not applicable
RMI III = U × M × CA-125 Cut off -200	U = 1 (0/ 1 parameter) U = 3 (≥2 parameters)	M = 1(premenopausal) M = 3(postmenopausal)	Not applicable
RMI IV = U × M × S × CA-125 Cut off -400	U = 1 (0 /1 parameter) U = 4 (≥2 parameters)	M = 1(premenopausal) M = 4(postmenopausal)	S = 1 (< 7 cm) S = 2 (≥7 cm)

- *Risk of malignancy algorithm(ROMA)*: Includes Ca 125, HE4 and menopausal status.
- *Risk of ovarian cancer algorithm (ROCA)*: Longitudinal assessment of Ca 125 and then risk stratification by doing a transvaginal sonography as a second step procedure.
- *International ovarian tumor analysis (IOTA) score*: Sensitivity 91.66%, Specificity 84.84% and accuracy of 88.88%.
- *Benign (B-rules)*: Unilocular cysts, smooth multi-locular tumor with largest diameter <100 mm, presence of solid components with largest diameter < 7 mm, presence of acoustic shadows and no blood flow on color Doppler.

- *Malignant (M-rules)*: Irregular solid tumors, irregular multi-locular solid tumor with largest diameter ≥100 mm, presence of ascites, at least four papillary (size > 3 mm) structures and very strong color flow in the tumor.
- *OVA-1*: Multi-analyte assay for risk stratification and it includes increased level of CA 125 and beta-2 microglobulin while decreased level of apolipoprotein A1, pre-albumin and transferrin levels in case of ovarian malignancy, A score greater than 5 in pre-menopausal and a score greater than 4.4 in post-menopausal is considered to be positive for malignancy.
- OVERA test includes apolipoprotein A-1, HE4, FSH, Transferrin and CA 125 levels.
- Surface-enhanced laser desorption/ionization-time of flight (SELDI-TOF) and Matrix-associated laser desorption/ionization-time of flight (MALDI-TOF)

Preinvasive Disease of Cervix

1. According to lower anogenital squamous terminology (LAST) nomenclature; cervical intraepithelial neoplasia-2 (CIN-2) can be divided into low grade and high grade by:

a. Ki-67 and p16
b. P53
c. HPV DNA
d. Colposcopy

2. The most common location of the original squamous columnar junction is:

a. Vaginal fornices
b. Ectocervix
c. Endocervix
d. None of the above

3. Transformation zone means the area between:

a. Internal os and external os
b. Histologic squamous columnar junction and original squamocolumnar junction (SCJ)
c. Histologic squamous columnar junction and new colposcopic squamocolumnar junction
d. Original squamous columnar junction and new colposcopic squamocolumnar junction

4. When the transformation zone is fully visible with the new SCJ on the ectocervix; it is known as:

a. Type I
b. Type II
c. Type III
d. None of the above

5. Major steps in the development of cervical cancer by human papillomavirus (HPV) include all, *except*:

a. Viral persistence
b. Progression
c. Clearance
d. Invasion

6. Reid's colposcopic index includes all, *except*:

a. Margin
b. Color
c. Vessels
d. Lesion size

(*N.B.:* Lesion size is included as an additional point in Swede's Colposcopic Index)

7. **Which is false about HPV?**
   a. Nonenveloped
   b. Double-stranded DNA
   c. RNA virus
   d. 72-sided icosahedral protein capsid

8. **E6 HPV oncoprotein includes all, *except*:**
   a. Binds and degrades host p53
   b. Increases telomerase activity in keratinocytes
   c. Binds with the *pRb* (retinoblastoma gene)
   d. Causes long-term infection and development of cancer

(*NB.*: E7 binds with *pRb*. Binding of E6 with p53 help bypass the HPV to bypass the cellular control mechanism of the host cells)

9. **E7 HPV oncoprotein causes all, *except*:**
   a. Binds with *pRb*
   b. Affects transition at G1/S phase of cell cycle
   c. Increases genomic instability
   d. E7 expression is an early event in malignant transformation

(Binding of E7 with *pRb*: makes the infected epithelial cells to produce new viral DNA and viral proteins)

10. **Prevalence of HPV in India is estimated to be up to:**
   a. 45%   b. 15%
   c. 60%   d. 70%

11. **Most frequently involved HPV in cervical cancer includes:**
   a. HPV 16   b. HPV 18
   c. HPV 31   d. HPV 11

12. **Which HPV types are associated with condylomata accuminata?**
   a. HPV 31 and HPV 33   b. HPV 45 and HPV 35
   c. HPV 16 and HPV 18   d. HPV 6 and HPV 11

13. **Which types of HPV is usually associated with adenocarcinoma of cervix?**
   a. HPV 16   b. HPV 18
   c. HPV 16 and HPV 18   d. HPV 45

14. **HPV testing is not recommended below age limit of:**
   a. 21 years   b. 25 years
   c. 40 years   d. 15 years

(*Note*: This is the new consensus recommendation of American Cancer Society 2020. Earlier it was 30 years of age for the start of primary testing or contesting of HPV)

15. **What screening method for cervical cancer is recommended below 25 years of age as per the new consensus of American Cancer Society 2020?**

a. Cytology
b. HPV testing
c. Both HPV and cytology
d. None of the above

16. **Between the age group of 30 and 65 years: Preferred cervical cancer screening method:**

a. Cotesting cytology and HPV testing every 5 years
b. Cotesting cytology and HPV testing every 3 years
c. Cytology every 3 yearly
d. HPV testing every yearly

17. **What is the recommended cervical screening method in a HPV-vaccinated lady?**

a. Only cytology
b. Only HPV testing
c. Same as an unvaccinated lady
d. No need of screening

18. **What is the recommended cervical screening method in a 66-year-old hysterectomized (done for benign indication) lady?**

a. Only cytology every 3 years
b. Only HPV testing every 5 years
c. No need of screening
d. Screening should be continued throughout her life

19. **Most common abnormal cervical cytology:**

a. ASC-US
b. HSIL
c. LSIL
d. ASC-H

20. **Strongest determining factor for viral persistence:**

a. Viral load
b. Host immunity
c. Sexual activity of the host
d. HPV type

21. **Percentage of CIN-3 progressing to invasive cancers over 30 years:**

a. 40%
b. 30%
c. 20%
d. 10%

22. **Established cofactors in HPV progression include all, *except*:**

a. Tobacco
b. Multiparity
c. Oral contraceptives (OCP) and barrier contraceptives
d. Age at first full term pregnancy
e. Host genetic factors

23. True about tobacco use and cervical carcinogenesis include all, *except*:
   a. Decreases the number of Langerhans cells in genital epithelium
   b. Mutagenic activity of genotoxic breakdown products in cervical secretions of smokers
   c. Is a strong risk factor for adenocarcinoma of cervix
   d. All of the above

24. Relative risk of invasive cervical cancer for first full-term pregnancy under 17 years compared with 25 years or older is:
   a. 4.77   b. 3.77
   c. 2.77   d. 1.77

25. Iatrogenic immunosuppression increases chances of CIN as compared to the general population by how many times?
   a. 4   b. 6
   c. 10   d. 16

26. HPV 16 and HPV 18 are responsible for how many percentage of total cervical cancers?
   a. 30%   b. 50%
   c. 70%   d. 90%

27. HPV 6 and HPV 11 are associated with what percentage of total anogenital warts?
   a. 90%   b. 70%
   c. 50%   d. 30%

28. True about HPV vaccine includes all, *except*:
   a. Virus like particle (VLP) technology
   b. DNA free VLP with no oncogenic potential
   c. Induces cell-mediated immunity in host
   d. Induces both cell-mediated and hormonal immunity in host

29. Quadrivalent vaccines protect against:
   a. HPV 16, 18, 6, and 11   b. HPV 16, 18, 31, and 35
   c. HPV 16, 18, 33, and 45   d. HPV 31, 33, 35, and 52

30. Cost effectiveness of HPV vaccines is not found in women over?
   a. 16 years   b. 26 years
   c. 36 years   d. 46 years
   (*NB*: Strategy for women over 26 years is "screen vaccinate")

31. Adjuvant in case of Gardasil is:
   a. Chloride   b. Magnesium
   c. Aluminum   d. Aluminum and bacterial lipid

32. Adjuvant (AS04) in case of Cervarix is:

a. Chloride
b. Magnesium
c. Aluminum
d. Aluminum and bacterial lipid

33. Approval of quadrivalent vaccination is in the age group of:

a. 16–26 years
b. 9–26 years
c. 9–16 years
d. 9–46 years

34. As per present studies the duration of protection after completion of HPV vaccination is up to:

a. 10 years
b. 8 years
c. 5 years
d. Lifelong

35. Efficacy of quadrivalent HPV vaccine against CIN II–III or adenocarcinoma in situ:

a. 70%
b. 80%
c. 90%
d. 99%

36. True about HPV vaccination includes all, *except*:

a. Therapeutic against pre-existing HPV vaccination
b. Category B Drug
c. Three doses
d. Between 9 and 26 years

37. False about HPV vaccine:

a. Demonstrated efficacy of 98–100%
b. Sustained efficacy for 10 years
c. Provide protection against other high-risk HPV types apart from HPV 16 to HPV 18
d. Therapeutic benefit in HPV infection

38. True about HPV vaccine includes all, *except*:

a. Vaccination of young sexually active women is beneficial
b. "Catch-up" vaccination till 26 years of age
c. Vaccinating boys provide herd immunity
d. Safe in pregnancy

39. Cotesting of LBC and HPV DNA should be done at intervals of:

a. 2 years
b. 3 years
c. 5 years
d. 6 years

40. Cytologic screening should not be done as per 2020 ASCCP guidelines before:

a. 21 years
b. 25 years
c. 26 years
d. 30 years

41. **LBC as a screening test should be done every:**

a. 1 year
b. 2 years
c. 3 years
d. 4 years

42. **Sensitivity of a single conventional pap smear:**

a. 51%
b. 61%
c. 71%
d. 81%

[Specificity of a single conventional pap smear is 66%]

43. **HPV DNA testing includes:**

a. Primary screening
b. Triage after LSIL/ASCUS
c. Test of cure following treatment of CIN-2 or CIN-3
d. All are correct

44. **Management of women with ASC-US includes:**

a. Repeat cytology
b. Immediate colposcopy
c. HPV DNA testing
d. All are correct

45. **Management of women with ASC-H and LSIL includes:**

a. Immediate colposcopy
b. Repeat cytology
c. HPV DNA testing
d. All are correct

46. **Ideal management for HSIL includes:**

a. Immediate loop electrosurgical excision
b. Immediate colposcopic examination
c. HPV DNA testing
d. a and b

47. **Work-up of women with atypical glandular cells:**

a. Colposcopy with endocervical sampling
b. HPV DNA testing
c. Endometrial sampling
d. All of the above

48. **For preinvasive cervical lesions; which among the following is considered as superior surgical technique?**

a. LEEP
b. Excisional conization
c. Cryosurgery
d. More research is needed for conclusion

49. **All are true about after treatment follow-up of CIN-2 and CIN-3, *except*:**

a. Cotesting at 12 months and 24 months after treatment
b. Routine screening should continue for at least 20 years
c. Routine screening may extend beyond 65 years of age
d. Routine screening should continue for at least next 10 years

50. Vaginal intraepithelial neoplasia 2 (VAIN 2) or VAIN 3 is most common in:

a. Upper one-third vagina
b. Middle one-third vagina
c. Lower one-third vagina
d. Lower one-third vagina

51. "Field effect" of squamous carcinogenesis is in the lower genital tract is more common with:

a. HPV 16
b. HPV 18
c. HPV 6
d. HPV 11

52. What percentage of VAIN 2 or VAIN 3 is HPV related?

a. 60%
b. 70%
c. 80%
d. 90%

53. What percentage of vaginal cancers is HPV related?

a. 60%
b. 70%
c. 80%
d. 90%

54. What percentage of VAIN has coexisting high-grade VIN?

a. 10%
b. 20%
c. 40%
d. 90%

55. HPV DNA can be detected in what percentage of vulval cancers?

a. 10%
b. 20%
c. 40%
d. 90%

56. Most common treatment of choice for VAIN:

a. 5% imiquimod cream
b. 5-fluorouracil
c. Cryosurgery
d. CO_2 laser

57. High-grade VIN is mainly due to:

a. HPV 16
b. HPV 18
c. HPV 31
d. HPV 35

58. Surveillance for recurrence of VIN should be for:

a. VAIN
b. CIN
c. VIN
d. PAIN

59. All are considered as specific region in the HPV viral genome, *except*:

a. Upstream regulatory region
b. Early region
c. Late region
d. Intermediate region

60. Noncoding region in the HPV genome includes:

a. Upstream regulatory region
b. Early region
c. Late region
d. None of the above

61. The region in the HPV genome that transcribes proteins and programs host cell to produce new viral DNA:

    a. Upstream regulatory protein   b. Early region
    c. Late region   d. None of the above

62. The region in the HPV genome that encodes for the capsid protein:

    a. Upstream regulatory protein   b. Early region
    c. Late region   d. None of the above

(*Note*: The late region in the open reading frame (ORF) L1 is similar in all HPV types while L2 is responsible for the different antigenicity of the different types of the HPV. The current HPV vaccines are targeted against the HPV capsid proteins and thus are HPV type specific.)

63. When compared to conventional pap smear; true about liquid-based cytology (LBC) are all, *except*:

    a. LBC reduces the rate of false negativity
    b. LBC lowers the specificity
    c. LBC increases the sensitivity
    d. LBC increases the true positivity
    e. All of the above

ANSWERS KEY

1. a	2. b	3. d	4. a	5. c	6. d	7. c
8. c	9. d	10. a	11. a	12. d	13. c	14. b
15. d	16. a	17. c	18. c	19. a	20. d	21. b
22. e	23. c	24. d	25. d	26. c	27. a	28. c
29. a	30. b	31. c	32. d	33. c	34. b	35. d
36. a	37. d	38. d	39. c	40. b	41. c	42. a
43. d	44. d	45. a	46. d	47. d	48. d	49. d
50. a	51. a	52. d	53. b	54. a	55. c	56. d
57. a	58. c	59. d	60. a	61. b	62. c	63. e

NOTES: PREINVASIVE DISEASE OF CERVIX

- Dysplasia is a lesion in which part of the epithelium has been replaced by cells showing varying degrees of atypia.
- Richart proposed the term cervical intraepithelial neoplasia (CIN) in 1973.
- Cervical intraepithelial neoplasia-3 is the most certain histologic surrogate marker of cancer risk.
- Cervical intraepithelial neoplasia-2 has the poorest interobserver reproducibility of any cervical histologic diagnosis. CIN 2 is a mixture of CIN 1 (infective phase) and CIN 3 (precancer phase). There is considerable heterogenicity in the clinical behavior, biology, and microscopic diagnosis of CIN 2 lesions.
- Infection with oncogenic human papillomavirus (HPV) types is strongly predictive of future risk of high-grade abnormalities.
- Low-grade squamous intraepithelial lesions (LSIL) should be managed conservatively by observation without treatment with an expectation of regression within 2 years. HSIL, particularly CIN 3, should be treated primarily by electrosurgical excision.
- *At 18–20 weeks of gestational age*: Columnar epithelial cells lining the vaginal tube is colonized by the upward growth of stratified squamous epithelium derived from the cloacal endoderm.
- The position of the original squamocolumnar junction in an infant is variable—ectocervix in 66%, endocervical canal in 30%, and vaginal fornices in 4%.
- The dynamic new squamocolumnar junction is called the colposcopic junction. The transformation zone is defined as that area lying between the original squamocolumnar junction and the colposcopic new squamocolumnar junction.
- Squamous metaplasia occurring in the transformation zone is a continuous process. Cervical neoplasia almost invariably originates within the transformation zone (TZ).
- The sensitivity of colposcopy for detecting prevailing precancerous lesions is around 50%. Colposcopic-guided biopsy can improve the detection rate.
- Human papillomavirus 16 lesions are the most visible colposcopic lesions.
- *Abnormal colposcopic findings (low-grade features)*: Acetowhite areas appear to be thin/translucent, rapidly fading, fine mosaic, fine punctation, irregular geographic border, and condylomatous/raised/papillary/flat areas
- *Abnormal colposcopic findings (high-grade features)*: Acetowhite areas appear to be thick dense, rapidly appearing/slowly fading, cuffed crypt

openings, variegated red and white, coarse mosaic/punctation, sharp border, ridge sign, peeling edges, and flat contour.

- *Abnormal colposcopic findings (invasive cancer suspicion)*: Atypical vessels, irregular surface, exophytic lesions, necrosis, and ulceration.
- Strength of acetoacetic solution is 3–5%.
- Strength of Lugol's iodine is 25% and application in cervix is known by "Schiller's test".
- *Reid Colposcopic Index*:

Reid's Colposcopic sign	0 point	1 point	2 points
Margin	Lesions are of exophytic condylomas distinct edges scalloped edges Satellite areas outside TZ	Lesions are regular shape	Lesions are rolled edges peeling edges
Color	Areas of faint whitening Shinny snow-white color	Shinny but gray-white color	Dull reflectance Oyster white color
Vessels	Fine caliber vessels and poorly formed patterns	No surface vessels	Definitive coarse punctation or Mosaic patterns
Iodine	Mahogany brown/ Mustard yellow but minor lesions with other above criteria	Partial Iodine staining (mottled appearance)	Mustard yellow staining with 3 or more points by the other above criteria
Scores of 0–2: Low-grade lesions		Scores of 6–8: High-grade lesions	

- Swede Colposcopic Index (Strander et al.):

Swede Score	0	1	2
Aceto uptake	Zero or transparent	Shady, milky neither transparent nor opaque	Distinct opaque White
Margins/ surface	Diffuse	Sharp but irregular jagged geographic satellites	Sharp even difference in surface level includes cuffing
Vessels	Fine and regular	Absent	Coarse or atypical
Lesion size	<5 mm	5–15 mm or 2 quadrants	>15 mm or 3–4 quadrants or undefined endocervical
Iodine staining	Brown	Faintly or patchy yellow	Distinct yellow

- Anogenital HPV types:

Low-risk types	6, 11, 26, 40, 42, 43, 44, 45, 53, 54, 61, 68, 72, 73, 81, 82
High-risk types	16, 18, 31, 33, 35, 39, 45, 51, 52, 56, 58, 59
High-risk possibility	66

- E6 and E7 are the primary HPV oncoproteins with numerous cellular targets.
- E6 proteins of the high-risk HPV types bind the tumor suppressor protein p53. This destroys the p53 and thus remove the p53 control of the host cell cycle. E6 also acts by increasing the telomerase activity (hTERT via c-myc).
- E7 is a primary transforming protein that binds with the retinoblastoma gene (*pRb*).
- E6 and E7 of low-risk HPV types only weakly bind p53 and *pRb* and thus do not immortalize keratinocytes in vitro.
- Usually sexually active women are exposed to HPV infection, but the HPV infection gets cleared within 2 years in most of the cases.
- Secondary peaks of HPV infection in some populations of older postmenopausal women may be due to reactivation of a latent viral reservoir and decrease in cell-mediated immunity.
- Human papillomavirus type is the strongest risk factor of viral persistence.
- High viral loads do not generally imply an increased risk of progression, except for HPV 16.
- Viral load measurement is not clinically important.
- The median time from HPV infection to CIN 3 is short. About 30% of cases of CIN 3 will progress to invasive cancer over 30 years.
- Cofactors in the progression of HPV infection—cigarette smoking, high parity, oral contraceptives (OCP), and immunosuppression.
- Human papillomavirus vaccine uses the virus-like particle (VLP) technology:
  - *Cervarix*: HPV 16 and HPV 18
  - *Gardasil*: HPV 6, 11, 16, and 18
  - *Gardasil 9*: HPV 6 ,11, 16, 18, 31, 33, 45, 52, and 58
- Inclusion of young males in HPV vaccination program is associated with a low return on investment especially when the coverage in females is >50% as this only increases the herd immunity induced protection to males. Most of the HPV-induced cancers in males are due to HPV-16. Vaccination above 26 years age group is not cost-effective.
- The vaccine-induced antibody is much higher than the immunity provided by the natural infection and sustained efficacy remain for about 10 years. For age <15 years, a dose vaccine of any HPV vaccine types is now validated and three doses for others. Vaccination may be started from 9 years and be given up to 26 years. Vaccination prior to sexual activity can provide the greatest public benefit.

- World Health Organization (WHO) Global "90/70/90" targets by 2030 mean: 90% of young adolescent that will be vaccinated, 70% women will be screened with HPV at least twice in their lifetime and 90% of women requiring it will be effectively treated for precancer or cancer. The draft threshold for cervical cancer elimination is four cases of cervical cancer per 100,000 women per annum.
- It is said that even one round of screening can substantially reduce an unscreened woman's risk of cervical cancer over her lifetime by around 41% if it has occurred at age 30 or 40.
- A positive HPV 16/18 test result should be followed by a colposcopic examination.
- The main benefit of HPV test in the screening strategy is the power of a negative result.

New Consensus of American Cancer Society 2020

- Over the years, major changes have included an older age to begin screening, discarding reference to first vaginal intercourse as a factor in beginning screening early, lengthening the screening interval, and the inclusion of HPV testing in screening protocols.
- Individuals with a cervix initiate cervical cancer screening at age 25 years and undergo primary human papillomavirus (HPV) testing every 5 years through age 65 years (preferred); if primary HPV testing is not available, then individuals aged 25–65 years should be screened with cotesting (HPV testing in combination with cytology) every 5 years or cytology alone every 3 years.
- On the basis of the consistent low cervical cancer incidence and mortality among women aged <25 years, the high incidence of transient infections, the risk of adverse obstetric outcomes of treatment, and the decision analysis demonstrating a favorable benefit-to-harm balance for beginning screening at age 25 years.
- Individuals aged >65 years who have no history of cervical intraepithelial neoplasia grade 2 or more severe disease within the past 25 years, and who have documented adequate negative prior screening in the prior 10 years, can discontinue all cervical cancer screening.
- These new screening recommendations differ in four important respects compared with the 2012 recommendations:
  - The preferred screening strategy is primary HPV testing every 5 years with cotesting or cytology.
  - The recommended age to start screening is 25 years rather than 21 years.
  - Primary HPV testing, as well as cotesting or cytology alone when primary testing is not available, is recommended starting at the age of 25 years rather than age of 30 years.

- The guideline is transitional (options for screening with cotesting or cytology alone are provided but should be phased out once full access to primary HPV testing for cervical cancer screening is available without barriers).
- Adequate negative prior screening is currently defined as two consecutive negative HPV tests, or two consecutive negative cotests, or three consecutive negative cytology tests within the past 10 years with the most recent test occurring within the recommended interval for the test used.
- These criteria do not apply to individuals who are currently under surveillance for abnormal screening results.
- Individuals older than age 65 years without conditions limiting life expectancy for whom sufficient documentation of prior screening is not available should be screened until criteria for screening cessation are met.
- Cervical cancer screening may be discontinued in individuals of any age with limited life expectancy.
- *Primary HPV test A test*: Detection of the DNA of oncogenic (high-risk) types of HPV in a sample taken from the cervix:
  - Cobas® HPV (approved 2014) HPV types 16 and 18
  - Onclarity™ HPV (approved 2018) HPV types 16, 18, 45, 31, 51, 52, 33+58, 35+39+68, and 56+59+66
- *Cotest (cytology and HPV test administered together)*: A test that combines cytology to look at cells under a microscope and test for HPV DNA in the same sample taken from the cervix:
  - Digene HC2
  - Cervista HPV HR
  - Cervista HPV16/18
  - Aptima HPV
  - Aptima HPV16 and 18/45
  - Cobas HPV (approved 2011) HPV types 16 and 18
  - Onclarity HPV (approved 2018) HPV types 16, 18, 45, 31, 51, 52, 33+58, 35+39+68, and 56+59+66.
- Self-sampling is a promising model of HPV DNA or RNA testing and has the potential of being very cost-effective method of cervical cancer screening. Till date, this method has not been approved as a validated tool of screening outside research activities.
- Dual stain testing (For p16 and Ki-67) in pap smear sample has emerged as a new way to more accurately predict pre-cancerous lesions in a HPV positive patient.
- *Triple test:* Pap smear + HPV test + Digital Cervicography. Optical imaging using artificial intelligence is coming up as a new method of screening but scientific validity.

Gestational Trophoblastic Neoplasia

1. Placental site trophoblastic tumor and epithelioid trophoblastic tumor originate from:

a. Cytotrophoblasts of villous trophoblast
b. Syncytiotrophoblasts of villous trophoblast
c. Intermediate cells of extra-villous trophoblast
d. None of the above

2. Characteristic "prune juice" vaginal bleeding is associated with:

a. Molar pregnancy
b. Abortion
c. Malignancy
d. None of the above

3. Pre-eclampsia is associated with molar pregnancy in:

a. 7%
b. 17%
c. 27%
d. 37%

4. Hyperthyroidism is associated with molar pregnancy in:

a. 7%
b. 17%
c. 27%
d. 37%

5. Theca luteal cysts > 6 cm diameter develop in about what percentage of molar pregnancy?

a. 50%
b. 40%
c. 30%
d. 20%

6. Familial recurrent molar pregnancy is associated with mutation of:

a. *NLRP7* gene in chromosome 19
b. *NLPR7* gene in chromosome 9
c. *NRPL7* gene in chromosome 13
d. *NPRL7* gene in chromosome 17

7. p57 is absent in:

a. Normal pregnancy
b. Complete mole
c. Partial mole
d. None of the above

8. After a molar suction evacuation; percentrage of local uterine invasion may occur in:

a. 4%
b. 10%
c. 15%
d. 20%

9. After a molar suction evacuation; percentage of choriocarcinoma may occur in:

a. 4%
b. 10%
c. 15%
d. 20%

10. Percentage of partial molar pregnancy developing into persistent postmolar tumor [gestational trophoblastic disease (GTD)]:

a. 2–4%
b. 8–10%
c. 12–14%
d. 16–18%

11. High risks for persistent postmolar tumor are seen in all, *except*:

a. hCG > 100,000 mIU/mL
b. Excessive uterine enlargement > 20 weeks
c. Theca luteal cyst > 6 cm diameter
d. Age < 40 years

12. Normal level of β-gonadotropin (β-hCG):

a. <2 mIU/mL
b. <5 mIU/mL
c. <7 mIU/mL
d. <10 mIU/mL

13. Chances of lung metastasis in choriocarcinoma:

a. 10%
b. 20%
c. 30%
d. 80%

14. Chances of vaginal metastasis in choriocarcinoma:

a. 10%
b. 20%
c. 30%
d. 80%

15. Chances of pelvic metastasis in choriocarcinoma:

a. 10%
b. 20%
c. 30%
d. 80%

16. Chances of brain metastasis in choriocarcinoma:

a. 10%
b. 20%
c. 30%
d. 80%

17. Chances of hepatic metastasis in choriocarcinoma:

a. 10%
b. 20%
c. 30%
d. 80%

18. What is the International Federation of Gynecology and Obstetrics (FIGO) staging of gestational trophoblastic neoplasia (GTN) when it spreads to the lung with/without known genital tract malignancies?

a. Stage I
b. Stage II
c. Stage III
d. Stage IV

19. In GTN, a patient is considered to be high risk and is considered for chemotherapy when the prognostic score is:

a. >5
b. >7
c. >8
d) >10

20. Diagnosis of postmolar GTN is based on all, *except*:

a. A plateau in β-hCG levels over at least 3 weeks
b. A 15% or greater rise in β-hCG levels for three or more values over at least 2 weeks
c. A 10% or greater rise in β-hCG levels for three or more values over at least 2 weeks
d. Evidence of metastasis or histological diagnosis of choriocarcinoma
e. Persistence of β-hCG levels 6 months after molar evacuation

21. Primary treatment of choice in placental site trophoblastic tumor (PSTT) or epithelial trophoblastic tumor (ETT):

a. Hysterectomy
b. Chemotherapy
c. Suction and evacuation
d. Radiotherapy

22. Follow-up in a patient of GTN stage I includes all, *except*:

a. Weekly β-hCG levels until they are normal for 3 consecutive weeks
b. Monthly β-hCG levels until they are normal for 12 consecutive months
c. Monthly β-hCG levels until they are normal for 24 consecutive months
d. None of the above

23. Follow-up in a patient of GTN stage II/stage III includes all, *except*:

a. Weekly β-hCG levels until they are normal for 3 consecutive weeks
b. Monthly β-hCG levels until they are normal for 12 consecutive months
c. Monthly β-hCG levels until they are normal for 24 consecutive months
d. None of the above

24. Follow-up in a patient of GTN stage IV includes all, *except*:

a. Weekly β-hCG levels until they are normal for 3 consecutive weeks
b. Monthly β-hCG levels until they are normal for 12 consecutive months
c. Monthly β-hCG levels until they are normal for 24 consecutive months
d. None of the above

25. True about oral contraceptive pills in GTN follow-up are all, *except*:

a. Contraception
b. Prevent cross-reactivity of endogenous luteinizing hormone (LH) and follicle-stimulating hormone (FSH) with β-hCG

    c. Should be given during the complete period of β-hCG testing

    d. Acts as a chemoprotective agent

26. **True about an adequate response in low risk nonmetastatic GTN after methotrexate as chemotherapy includes all, *except*:**

    a. Fall in β-hCG level by 1 log after a single course of chemotherapy

    b. Resistant is considered when there is failure of two consecutive courses of methotrexate and should converted into actinomycin D

    c. Resistant is considered when there is failure of three consecutive courses of methotrexate and should be converted into EMA-CO regime

    d. When both methotrexate and actinomycin D fail in response; then only should start EMA-CO in such cases

27. **Increased risk of second malignancy is associated with:**

    a. Actinomycin D   b. Vincristine

    c. Cyclophosphamide   d. Etoposide

28. **Which is the most common karyotype in complete mole:**

    a. 46 XX   b. 46 XY

    c. 69 XXY   d. 69 XYY

29. **Ratio of the percentage of free β-hCG to free α-hCG in complete mole is:**

    a. 20.9   b. 2.4

    c. 40.9   d. 2.8

30. **Ratio of the percentage of free β-hCG to free α-hCG in partial mole is:**

    a. 20.9   b. 2.4

    c. 40.9   d. 2.8

31. **Phantom hCG is due to presence of:**

    a. LH

    b. Heterophile antibodies

    c. Hyperglycosylated hCG

    d. Thyroid-stimulating hormone (TSH)

32. **Quiescent GTN is due to absence of:**

    a. LH   b. Heterophile hCG

    c. Hyperglycosylated hCG   d. TSH

33. **True about PSTT includes all, *except*:**

    a. Negative for p63

    b. Positive for p63

    c. Diffusely positive for cytokeratin

    d. Diffusely positive for inhibin A

34. **Gestational trophoblastic neoplasia which has got high propensity for lymphatic spread:**
a. Epithelioid trophoblastic tumor
b. Placental site trophoblastic tumor
c. Choriocarcinoma
d. No lymphatic spread in GTN

35. **Reasons for treatment failure in case of GTN:**
a. Use of single agent computed tomography (CT) for patients with high-risk disease
b. Inappropriate use of weekly intramuscular dose of methotrexate or pulse-dose IV infusion methotrexate
c. Delay in referrals to oncology centers after failure of single agent chemotherapy
d. All of the above

36. **"Hook-effect" of ELISA serum hCG:**
a. Very high levels of serum hCG
b. Very low level of serum hCG
c. Unstable hCG
d. Stable hCG

37. **Epithelioid trophoblastic tumor and placental site nodule (PSN) can be differentiated by:**
a. Cyclin E (negative in ETT)
b. Cyclin E (highly positive in ETT)
c. Cyclin E (highly positive in PSN)
d. Cyclin E (negative in PSN)

38. **False as per the National Comprehensive Cancer Network (NCCN) guidelines for GTN:**
a. Imaging is required during follow-up after normalization of β-hCG for postmolar GTN or choriocarcinoma
b. Imaging is not required during follow-up after normalization of β-hCG for postmolar GTN or choriocarcinoma
c. Imaging is required in case of PSTT and ETT follow-up
d. Depends upon the prognostic scoring

39. **Prognostic scoring system is not valid for:**
a. PSTT
b. ETT
c. Both PSTT and ETT
d. Valid for all types of GTN

40. **Human chorionic gonadotropin (hCG) plateau during treatment of GTN is defined as:**
a. <10% decrease in hCG over two treatment cycles (4 weeks in total)
b. <15% decrease in hCG over two treatment cycles (4 weeks in total)
c. <10% decrease in hCG over three treatment cycles (6 weeks in total)
d. <15% decrease in hCG over three treatment cycles (6 weeks in total)

41. **True about chemotherapy regimes in GTN:**

a. Continued until 2–3 full cycles past normalization of hCG
b. Continues until 3–4 full cycles past normalization of hCG
c. Continued until 2–3 full cycles past normalization of imaging and hCG
d. Continued until 3–4 full cycles past normalization of imaging and hCG

42. **Recommendation about oophorectomy during hysterectomy for GTN:**

a. Should always be done concurrently
b. Should never be done unless other disease pathology in ovaries
c. Should be done when theca luteal cysts are >6 cm diameter
d. Cystectomy for theca luteal cysts should be done

43. **Poor prognostic marker for PSTT includes all, *except*:**

a. >5/10 mitotic count per high-power field
b. Deep myometrial invasion
c. Extensive coagulative necrosis
d. Interval since last index pregnancy >2 years
e. Lymphovascular space invasion is not a prognostic factor

44. **As per NCCN guidelines:**

a. Methotrexate 30–50 mg/m^2 IM weekly or methotrexate infusion 300 mg/m^2 due to lesser efficacy
b. Pulse actinomycin-D should not be used as secondary therapy for methotrexate resistant disease nor as primary therapy for choriocarcinoma
c. *In patients with widely metastatic disease (prognostic score > 12):* Low-dose induction chemotherapy with etoposide 100 mg/m^2/day IV and cisplatin 20 mg/m^2/day IV on day 1 and day 2 every 7 days for 1–3 courses prior to start of EMA-CO or EMA-EP
d. Use of granocyte-colony stimulating factor (G-CSF) as primary prophylaxis with etoposide/cisplatin or etoposide/carboplatin
e. All of the above

45. **The incidences of pelvic lymph node metastasis in PSTT/ETT in stage I tumor:**

a. 1–2%
b. 2–5%
c. 5–10%
d. 5–15%

46. **True about poor response to initial single agent chemotherapy and switch from single agent to EMA-CO is all, *except*:**

a. hCG level plateaus (<10% change) for two treatment cycles (4 weeks)
b. hCG level rises (>10% change) for one treatment cycle (2 weeks)
c. hCG level plateaus (<15% change) for two treatment cycles (4 weeks)
d. Repeat metastatic work up should be done

ANSWERS KEY

1. c	2. a	3. c	4. a	5. a	6. a	7. b
8. c	9. a	10. a	11. d	12. b	13. d	14. c
15. b	16. a	17. a	18. c	19. b	20. b	21. a
22. c	23. c	24. b	25. d	26. c	27. d	28. a
29. a	30. b	31. b	32. c	33. b	34. b	35. d
36. a	37. b	38. b	39. c	40. a	41. a	42. b
43. e	44. e	45. d	46. c			

NOTES: GESTATIONAL TROPHOBLASTIC NEOPLASIA

- Classification of gestational trophoblastic disease:
  - Complete hydatidiform mole
  - Partial hydatidiform mole $\Big\}$ (80% of GTD)
  - Invasive mole (nonmetastatic GTN) (15% of GTD)
  - Choriocarcinoma (metastatic GTN)
  - Placental site trophoblastic tumor (metastatic GTN $\Big\}$ (5% of GTD)
  - Epithelioid trophoblastic tumor (metastatic GTN)
- Intermediate trophoblastic tumors (ITT) comprises PSTT and ETT. They are very rare and incidence is about one in 100,000 pregnancies.
- Postmolar GTN:
  - Human chorionic gonadotropin levels plateau for four consecutive values over 3 weeks
  - Human chorionic gonadotropin levels rise $\geq 10\%$ for three values over 2 weeks
  - Human chorionic gonadotropin persistence 6 months after molar evacuation
  - Histopathological diagnosis of choriocarcinoma $\pm$ metastatic disease
- Weekly intramuscular or pulse-dose IV infusion methotrexate is no longer recommended.
- Regimes for low-risk GTN:
  - Methotrexate
    0.4 mg/kg/day (maximum 25 mg/day) IV or IM daily × 5 days. Repeat every 14 days OR
    1 mg/kg IM every other day × 4 days (days 1, 3, 5, and 7). Alternating every other day with leucovorin 0.1 mg/kg round up to the nearest

5 mg dose increment or 15 mg poor IM 30 hours after each methotrexate dose on days 2, 4, 6, and 8. Repeat every 14 days.
  - Dactinomycin
    10–12 µg/kg (0.5 mg dose) IV daily × 5 days. Repeat every 14 days OR 1.25 mg/m^2 (maximum 2 mg) IV pulse. Repeat every 14 days.
- Regimes for high-risk GTN: EMA-CO:
  - Etoposide 100 mg/m^2/day IV on day 1 and 2
  - Dactinomycin 0.5 mg IV push on day 1 and 2
  - Methotrexate 300 mg/m^2 iv infusion over 12 hours on Day 1 or Methotrexate 100 mg/m^2 iv push followed by 200 mg/m^2 iv infusion over 12 hours
  - Leucovorin 15 mg PO or IM every 12 hours for four doses starting 24 hours after the start of methotrexate infusion
  - Cyclophosphamide 600 mg/m^2 IV on day 8
  - Vincristine 1 mg/m^2 (maximum 2 mg) IV over 5–10 minutes on day 8
  - Repeat every 2 weeks until hCG normalizes and then continue for an additional 6–8 weeks.
  - Low-dose chemotherapy with etoposide 100 mg/m^2/day IV and cisplatin 20 mg/m^2/day IV on days 1 and 2 every 7 days for 1–3 courses prior to starting EMA-Co in patients with prognostic score >12 (because of significant changes of bleeds from these metastases due to chemotherapy).
  - Filgrastim 300 µg subcutaneously on days 9–14 of each EMA-CO cycle
  - For those who are not responding well to EMA-CO: EMA-EP (etoposide-methotrexate-actinomycin-D/etoposide-cisplatin) or EP-EMA regime is preferred.
- For methotrexate resistant GTN:
  - EMA-CO
  - TP/TE (paclitaxel-cisplatin/paclitaxel-etoposide)
  - BEP (bleomycin-etoposide-cisplatin)
  - VIP (etoposide-ifosfamide-cisplatin)
  - ICE (ifosfamide-carboplatin-etoposide)
  - TIP (paclitaxel-ifosfamide-cisplatin)
  - *Others*: 5-FU, capecitabine, gemcitabine, pembrolizumab, nivolumab
- For intermediate trophoblastic tumor (PSTT and ETT)
  - EMA/EP or EP/EMA
  - Other regimes are TP/TE, BEP, VIP, and ICE
- Second-line/Salvage Therapy (Relapse after EMA-CO)
  - EMA-EP (Etoposide/Methotrexate/Actinomycin- Etoposide/Cisplatin)
- Prophylactic chemotherapy at the time of a complete molar evacuation is controversial and is usually offered to high-risk complete molar pregnancy patients when the hormonal follow-up is unavailable or unreliable.
- *Human chorionic gonadotropins*: Human chorionic gonadotropins is a disease specific tumor marker of gestational trophoblastic disease

and can be measured in the blood and urine. hCG is produced by syncytiotrophoblasts and is maximum of 60,000 to 80,000 mIU/mL at 10 weeks period of gestation and then declines to around 12,000 mIU/mL during the reminder of pregnancy. It has two subunits; namely nonspecific α-subunit and specific β-subunit. hCG molecules produced by the trophoblastic tumor are more heterogenous and several forms are available. The various fragments of hCG molecules in GTD are hyperglycosylated, nicked, C-terminal truncated β-subunit, nicked free β-subunit and a free α-subunit. In follow-up of GTD, we thus measure the total quantitative value of hCG including its various degradation molecules.

Hyperglycosylated hCG is produced by cytotrophoblasts in early part of gestation and is a reflection of the trophoblastic invasion of the implantation site and feto-maternal circulation. It is further produced in malignant trophoblastic tissues and indicates invasion.

False positive or "phantom hCG" is due to the presence of non-specific heterophile antibodies that mimic hCG and is present in 3–4% of normal patients. As these heterophile antibodies do not pass through the urine because of their large molecular size; they are absent in urine. Also, serial dilution of the serum sample would not show a decrease in the detected antibody. As the α-subunit of hCG cross reacts with the FSH, LH, TSH and this can lead to false elevation of the total hCG level. hCG normally increases with age and thus may be falsely elevated in a nonpregnant perimenopausal woman or in a postmenopausal woman. To avoid such confusions, women may be offered oral contraceptive to suppress the endogenous LH and FSH and then simultaneous test of hCG, FSH, and LH can be done for a correct evaluation of the total hCG.

Apart from the false positive hCG; there lies another entity named as "Quiescent GTD". It is a low level of consistent hCG which is detectable after an abortion or GTD but without any presence of disease activity. There is no detectable level of any hyperglycosylated hCG. This low level of hCG is produced by individual or disperse foci of trophoblastic tissues without any invasive potential. This Quiescent hCG may progress to active GTN in approximately 30% cases.

- Partial Mole stains positive for p57kip2 (also positive by hydropic abortus) and PHLDA2.
- hCG level > 100,000 mIU/mL are seen in only 10% of patients with partial moles.
- FISH can be used to distinguish between a p57kip2 positive partial mole (triploid) and hydropic abortus (diploid).
- Germline mutations in *NLRP7* and *KHDC3L* are observed respectively in 48–80% and 10–14% of patients with repetitive moles. Assisted reproduction techniques with the use of donor eggs are recommended for future pregnancies if such mutations are identified.

- *Placental site trophoblastic tumor*: Absence of villi and low mitotic counts. Presence of intermediate trophoblastic without syncytiotrophoblastic tissues (low secretion of beta-hCG). They stain positively for human placental lactogen and diffusely positive for Mel-CAM and cytokeratin. Serum free β-hCG subunit may be a marker for this disease.
- *Epithelioid trophoblastic tumor*: Also derived from intermediate trophoblastic tissues and show strong expression of p63. Presence of hyaline-like matrix and extensive necrosis are detected. Epithelioid trophoblastic tumors can be misdiagnosed as a squamous carcinoma.
- Minimally aggressive GTN is a chemo-refractory type of GTN characterised by a slow growth rate and low levels of hyperglycosylated hCG.

Cervical Cancer

1. Screening for carcinogenic human papillomavirus (HPV) is an example of:

a. Secondary screening
b. Primary screening
c. Tertiary screening
d. Both primary and secondary screening

2. Pap smear screening is an example of:

a. Secondary screening
b. Primary screening
c. Tertiary screening
d. None of the above

3. False negative rate for pap smears in invasive cancer cervix may be up to:

a. 10%
b. 20%
c. 40%
d. 50%

4. In cancer cervix, which is the most common site of occult metastasis?

a. Parametrium
b. Peritoneum
c. Omentum
d. Pelvic and para-aortic lymph nodes (LNs)

5. False positive LNs on computed tomography (CT) scan can be due to all, *except*:

a. Inflammatory changes
b. Hyperplastic changes
c. Infective changes
d. Microscopic deposits

6. Computed tomography scan accuracy of detecting para-aortic LN is approximately:

a. 85%
b. 50%
c. 75%
d. 95%

(*Note:* Same question on false negative rate is 13% and false positive rate is 21%.)

7. Accuracy of magnetic resonance imaging (MRI) for tumor size in cancer cervix is:

a. 83%

b. 73%

c. 93%

d. 99%

8. Accuracy of MRI for depth of stromal invasion in cancer cervix is:

a. 68%

b. 78%

c. 88%

d. 98%

9. For disease stage evaluation in cervical cancer; MRI has an accuracy of:

a. 100%

b. 90%

c. 80%

d. 70%

(*Note:* Accuracy of CT scan 65%)

10. Fluorodeoxyglucose-positron emission tomography (FDG-PET) scan for para-aortic LN metastasis in cancer cervix has a specificity of:

a. 75%

b. 85%

c. 95%

d. 100%

(*Note:* Same question on sensitivity is 84%)

11. Range of accuracy for abdominopelvic LN by fine needle aspiration cytology (FNAC) in cervical cervix is:

a. 74–95%

b. 65–74%

c. 84–95%

d. 74–85%

12. Ovarian involvement in cancer cervix is through:

a. Hematogenous

b. Direct extension

c. Lymphatic spread

d. Retrograde lymphovascular space invasion (LVSI) and neuronal spread

13. Microinvasive disease is up to (as per International Federation of Gynecology and Obstetrics FIGO):

a. Stage I A1 and stage I A2

b. Stage I A1 only

c. Stage I A1 and LVSI

d. Stage I A1, stage I A2, and LVSI

14. Fertility preserving surgery in a stage I A2 should not ideally be:

a. Cone biopsy plus pelvic LN dissection

b. Radical trachelectomy ± pelvic LN dissection

c. Only cone biopsy

d. None of the above

(*Note*: Only cone biopsy up to stage I A1)

15. True about fertility-sparing surgery in cancer cervix includes all, *except*:

a. Small cell neuroendocrine type Ca cervix
b. Endocervical curettage should be a part of the procedure
c. Lesion size <2 cm
d. Cone biopsy should have a negative margin of 3 mm and nonfragmented

16. True about fertility-sparing surgery in cancer cervix includes all, *except*:

a. Adenoma malignum or minimal deviation adenocarcinoma
b. Endocervical curettage should be a part of the procedure
c. Lesion size <2 cm
d. Cone biopsy should have a negative margin of 3 mm and nonfragmented

17. Chances of lymphatic metastasis in microinvasive disease (FIGO Stage I A1 without LVSI) are:

a. 1%   b. 2%
c. 3%   d. 4%

18. Permissible or ideal treatment strategy up to stage I A1 are all, *except*:

a. Cone biopsy if desires fertility
b. Extrafascial hysterectomy
c. Radical hysterectomy plus pelvic LN dissection
d. None of the above
(*Note:* Preferred cone biopsy is cold knife cone biopsy)

19. What is the most common side-effect of radical trachelectomy?

a. Recurrent candidiasis
b. Isthmic stenosis
c. Dysmenorrhea
d. Irregular menstruation

20. Sentinel lymph node (SLN) mapping in fertility preserving surgery should be included in all, *except*:

a. Stage I A1 with LVSI   b. Stage I B1
c. Stage I B2   d. Stage I A1 without LVSI

21. Ideal treatment for stage I A2 cancer cervix (squamous cell carcinoma or adenocarcinoma) is:

a. Modified radical hysterectomy plus pelvic LN dissection
b. Extrafascial hysterectomy
c. Intrafascial hysterectomy
d. Radical hysterectomy

22. **What is the distance between two skip lesions in multifocal cervical adenocarcinoma?**

a. 2 mm
b. 3 mm
c. 5 mm
d. 10 mm

23. **What is not true in case of stage I A1 lesions?**

a. Positive corelation between depth of invasion and presence of LVSI
b. Positive corelation between LN metastasis and presence of LVSI
c. Lymphovascular space invasion is uncommon in stage I A1
d. Cone biopsy can be a valid option

24. **Poor prognosticators of cancer cervix are all, *except*:**

a. Squamous cell carcinoma
b. Adenocarcinoma
c. Adenosquamous
d. Small cell carcinoma

25. **Ideal time to do a radical hysterectomy after a margin negative cone biopsy is:**

a. Immediately
b. After 3 weeks
c. After 6 weeks
d. After 8 weeks

(*Note:* In case of margin positive cone biopsy; recommendation is immediate radical hysterectomy after cone biopsy but there is increase in morbidity)

26. **Level 3 of LN dissection includes:**

a. External and internal iliac LN
b. Common Iliac including presacral LN
c. Aortic inframesenteric LN
d. Aortic infrarenal LN

(*Note:* Level 1: External and internal iliac LN; Level 2: Common iliac including presacral LN; Level 3: Aortic infrarenal LN)

27. **Type III radical hysterectomy is ideal for:**

a. Stage I A1
b. Stage I B
c. Stage I A2
d. None of the above

28. **Extended radical hysterectomy corresponds to which types of hysterectomy as per Piver et al.?**

a. Type III
b. Type IV
c. Type V
d. None of the above

29. **As per Querleu and Morrow (Kyoto classification); paracervical LNs means:**

a. Lymph nodes lateral to obturator nerve
b. Lymph nodes medial and caudal to the obturator nerve
c. Lymph nodes medial and cephaloid to the obturator nerve
d. Lymph nodes both medial and lateral to the obturator nerve

30. False negative rate of SLNs in cancer cervix is:

    a. 6.8%　　　　　　　　　　b. 8.6%
    c. 5%　　　　　　　　　　　d. 3%

31. Studies show that sentinel node mapping and ultrastaging in cancer cervix can give a false negative rate of:

    a. 1.3%　　　　　　　　　　b. 2.3%
    c. 3.3%　　　　　　　　　　d. 4.3%

32. Fertility preserving surgery in cancer cervix can be done up to:

    a. Stage I A1　　　　　　　　b. Stage I A2
    c. Stage I B1　　　　　　　　d. Stage I B2

33. Most common urinary bladder dysfunction after radical hysterectomy is:

    a. Hypotonic bladder dysfunction
    b. Hypertonic bladder dysfunction
    c. Mixed bladder dysfunction
    d. None of the above

34. Which of the following carries the worst prognosis after a radical hysterectomy?

    a. Hypotonic bladder dysfunction
    b. Hypertonic bladder dysfunction
    c. Mixed bladder dysfunction
    d. None of the above

35. Impaired fertility following radical trachelectomy is due to:

    a. Cervical stenosis
    b. Surgical adhesions
    c. Decreased cervical mucus production
    d. All of the above

36. True about radical trachelectomy are all, *except*:

    a. Increased first trimester abortion
    b. Increased second trimester abortion
    c. Overall recurrences rate is 3–6%
    d. Overall death rate is 2–5%

37. True about neoadjuvant chemotherapy (NACT) in cancer cervix are all, *except*:

    a. Surgery is difficult due to postchemotherapy inflammatory reactions
    b. Low complete pathologic response by NACT
    c. Prolongs treatment time (radiation therapy is given 6 weeks after radical hysterectomy)
    d. Contraindicated in pregnancy

38. Most cost-effective treatment of cancer cervix with a disease-free interval of 5-year survival of about 70% is:

a. Radical hysterectomy + pelvic lymphadenectomy + para-aortic lymphadenectomy and tailored concurrent chemoradiation therapy (CCRT)
b. Primary chemoradiation
c. Neoadjuvant chemotherapy followed by radical hysterectomy and tailored concurrent chemoradiation
d. All are equally cost-effective.

39. Major prognostic indicators for tailored concurrent chemoradiation includes all, *except*:

a. Positive LNs
b. Positive parametrial involvement
c. LVSI
d. Positive vaginal cuff margins

40. Sedlis prognostic criteria for tailored concurrent chemoradiation includes all, *except*:

a. Size of the lesion
b. Depth of stromal invasion
c. LVSI
d. Histology of the cell type

41. The Gynecologic Oncology Group (GOG) score for traditional concurrent chemoradiation after radical hysterectomy and pelvic lymphadenectomy includes all, *except*:

a. Size of the lesion
b. Depth of stromal invasion
c. LVSI
d. Histology of the cell types

42. Recurrence rate in cancer cervix at 3 years with a GOG score > 120 is about:

a. 20%
b. 30%
c. 40%
d. 50%

43. Close vaginal margin in a specimen of radical hysterectomy is defined as a distance between tumor from vaginal margin of resection is:

a. <0.8 cm
b. <0.5 cm
c. <1 cm
d. <2 cm

44. Most important prognostic factor in cancer cervix is:

a. Age of the patient
b. Histological types
c. Size of the lesion
d. Status of the LNs

45. 5-year survival with negative parametrium in a specimen of radical hysterectomy is about:

a. 85%
b. 95%
c. 75%
d. 65%

(*Note:* If parametrial invasion is present in radical hysterectomy specimen: 5-year survival is 62%)

46. **5-year survival in case of positive parametrial margin and positive lymph node is about:**

a. 69%
b. 79%
c. 52%
d. 39%

47. **Adenocarcinoma variant of Cancer cervix include all *except*:**

a. Disseminate more hematogenous
b. More radioresistant
c. Smoking is a risk factor
d. Obesity is a risk factor

(Adenocarcinoma Cancer Cervix: HPV 18 is more associated with it and there are higher chances of ovarian metastasis)

48. **True about prognostic factor in adenocarcinoma variant of cancer cervix includes all, *except*:**

a. HPV-18
b. Positive peritoneal cytology
c. Pretreatment CA125
d. Equal ovarian metastasis compared to squamous cell carcinoma variant

49. **Which is false about the association of adenoma malignum variant of cancer cervix?**

a. Very poor prognosis
b. Peutz–Jeghers syndrome
c. Sex-cord tumor
d. Pap smears usually normal or show minor abnormalities

50. **Early painful presentation is seen in which type of cell variant of cancer cervix?**

a. Glassy cell carcinoma
b. Small cell carcinoma
c. Adenoma malignum
d. Adenoid cystic carcinoma

51. **Good prognosis of cancer cervix includes all, *except*:**

a. Adenoid basal carcinoma
b. Adenoma malignum
c. Villoglandular papillary adenocarcinoma
d. Neuroendocrine carcinomas

52. **Diethylstilbestrol (DES) exposure is related to:**

a. Neuroendocrine carcinomas
b. Clear cell adenocarcinomas
c. Villoglandular papillary adenocarcinomas
d. Adenoid cystic carcinoma

53. **Villoglandular papillary adenocarcinoma of the cervix is associated with all, *except:***

a. Young age
b. Excellent prognosis
c. Uncommon variety
d. None of the above

54. **True about cervical lymphoma includes all, *except*:**

a. Diffuse large cell B-cell lymphoma is the most common type
b. Expanded cervix with no ulceration or fungation
c. Radical surgery is the treatment of choice
d. R-CHOP regime is given with good prognosis

55. **Rhabdomyosarcomas of cervix are associated with the following, *except*:**

a. Most common is the sarcoma botryoides variant
b. Pediatric age group
c. Presents as polypoidal vaginal mass
d. Carries a poor prognosis even with multimodal treatment

56. **Verrucous carcinoma of cervix includes all, *except*:**

a. Slow growing tumor
b. Locally aggressive papillomatous lesion
c. Radical surgery is the treatment
d. Primary radiation therapy is the treatment of choice

57. **Metastasis from any extragenital cancers occurs mostly to:**

a. Ovary
b. Vagina
c. Cervix
d. Endometrium

58. **Most commonly documented primary site metastasizing to cervix is:**

a. Stomach
b. Ovary
c. Colon
d. Breast

59. **Adverse prognostic factor after invasive cervix cancer found after simple hysterectomy include all, *except*:**

a. Hemoglobin < 10 gm
b. Interval between surgery and radiation longer than 80 days
c. Absence of brachytherapy
d. Interval between surgery and radiation longer than 56 days

60. **Monsel solution is:**

a. Ferric sulfate
b. Silver sulfate
c. Silver subsulfate
d. Ferric subsulfate

61. **Risk of central recurrences includes all, *except*:**

a. Status of LN
b. Size of the lesion
c. Parametrial involvement
d. Stage of the disease

62. **Least common side-effect of bevacizumab is:**

a. Hypertension
b. Thromboembolism
c. Anemia
d. Neutropenia

63. **During anterior exenteration; which of the following artery is not sacrificed:**

a. Internal pudendal artery
b. Inferior hemorrhoidal artery
c. Obturator artery
d. Vesical artery

64. **Clinical triad of pelvic wall extension of the disease includes all, *except*:**

a. Rectovaginal fistula
b. Unilateral leg edema
c. Sciatic pain
d. Ureteral obstruction

65. **It is generally accepted that the entire course of radiotherapy [external beam radiotherapy (EBRT) + brachytherapy] should be completed in:**

a. 8 weeks
b. 10 weeks
c. 12 weeks
d. No such time frame

66. **Most patients with cancer cervix in pregnancy are detected in:**

a. Stage I
b. Stage II
c. Stage III
d. Cannot be staged in pregnancy

67. **Ideally before start of pelvic radiation; ovarian transposition should be considered in [as mentioned in National Comprehensive Cancer Network (NCCN) guidelines]:**

a. Age <45 years and early staged disease
b. Age >45 years
c. Age <50 years
d. Young reproductive age in all stages

68. **As per NCCN guidelines all are true about ovarian transposition in cancer cervix, *except*:**

a. Age <45 years
b. Early stage
c. Squamous cell carcinoma
d. Adenocarcinoma variety

69. **True about point A (paracervical reference point) in cancer cervix radiation therapy:**

a. Most widely validated dosing parameter
b. Does not take into account the three-dimensional shape of the tumor
c. Does not take into account the individual tumor to normal tissue structure
d. All of the above

70. **Adjuvant radiation therapy in cancer cervix after radical surgery should be considered when:**

a. Positive LN
b. Parametrial infiltration
c. Positive vaginal cuff surgical margin
d. Any one of the above

71. **Sedlis criteria (intermediate risk factors) include all, *except*:**

a. Tumor size
b. LVSI
c. Depth of stromal invasion
d. Histology of cancer cervix

72. **Sedlis criteria include all, *except*:**

a. >1/3rd stromal invasion
b. Presence of LVSI
c. Cervical tumor diameter > 4 cm
d. Close vaginal margin

73. **Which is the preferred radio sensitizing agent in case of cancer cervix radiation therapy?**

a. Carboplatin
b. Cisplatin
c. Fluorouracil
d. None of the above

74. **When a posthysterectomy specimen meets two of Sedlis criteria; recommendation is:**

a. Observation
b. Brachytherapy
c. Pelvic EBRT
d. Pelvic EBRT with CCRT

75. **Recommendation when an incidental cervical cancer stage I A1 without LVSI detected after type I extra-fascial, hysterectomy is:**

a. Surveillance
b. EBRT
c. Brachytherapy
d. EBRT with CCRT + brachytherapy

76. **As per NCCN guidelines, the first line single agent chemotherapy option for recurrent or metastatic cervical cancer includes all, *except*:**

a. Cisplatin
b. Carboplatin
c. Paclitaxel
d. Bevacizumab

(Preferred is cisplatin as per NCCN)

77. **As per NCCN guidelines, preferred second line drug for treating PD-L1 positive or MSI-H/d MMR cervical cancer is:**

a. Pembrolizumab
b. Bevacizumab
c. Nab-paclitaxel
d. Topotecan

(Similarly for NTRK gene fusion positive cases: Larotrectinib or Entrectinib)

78. As per NCCN guidelines, preferred first line combination therapy in metastatic cervical cancer includes:

a. Cisplatin/paclitaxel
b. Cisplatin/paclitaxel/bevacizumab
c. Cisplatin/gemcitabine
d. Cisplatin/topotecan

79. Addition of bevacizumab to combination chemotherapy therapy in metastatic or recurrent cervical cancer causes all, *except*:

a. Significant improvement in overall survival
b. Decrease in quality-of-life
c. Increase in toxicity
d. Category 1 recommendation

80. Surveillance for a treated case of cancer cervix should be continued for:

a. 2 years
b. 3 years
c. 10 years
d. 20 years

81. Surveillance for a treated case of CIN III should be continued for:

a. 2 years
b. 3 years
c. 10 years
d. 20 years

82. All are true about NACT followed by surgery in treatment of cancer cervix, *except*:

a. No improvement in survival
b. Decreases the need of adjuvant radiation therapy
c. Response to NACT is a prognostic factor progression-free survival (PFS) and overall survival
d. Use is recommended outside clinical trials also

83. High-risk disease in a specimen of cancer cervix is considered in all, *except*:

a. Positive pelvic LNs
b. Positive surgical margin
c. Positive parametrium
d. Lymphovascular space invasion

84. Node-margin-parametrium negative should be offered adjuvant radiation therapy when:

a. One Sedlis criteria is present
b. Two Sedlis criteria is present
c. Three Sedlis criteria is present
d. Not relevant

85. Developing countries account for what percentage of total cervical cancer load?

a. 35%
b. 45%
c. 55%
d. 85%

86. Prevalence of HPV in countries with high incidence of cancer cervix is:

a. 5–10%
b. 10–20%
c. 50–60%
d. 60–70%

87. Squamous cell carcinoma accounts for what percentage of cancer cervix?

a. 50%
b. 60%
c. 70%
d. 80%

88. Adenocarcinoma accounts for what percentage of cancer cervix?

a. 20%
b. 30%
c. 40%
d. 50%

89. Increase incidences of adenocarcinoma worldwide is mainly due to:

a. Cervical cytologic screening is less effective for adenocarcinoma
b. Geographical disparities exist
c. HPV testing is ineffective in detection of cancer cervix
d. None of the above

90. Not a part of new revised 2018 FIGO staging for cancer cervix:

a. Lateral horizontal extent of the disease in Stage I A is not considered
b. Pelvic and para-aortic LN involvement is considered
c. Lesion size > 2 cm and ≤4 cm is considered
d. Involvement of lymphovascular spaces is considered

(Isolated tumor cells do not change the stage of the disease but their presence should be noted)

91. Not a part of new revised 2018 FIGO staging for cancer cervix:

a. Imaging
b. Pathology
c. Clinical
d. Tumor markers

92. Accepted criteria for microinvasive disease in cancer cervix are:

a. Up to stage I A1 with no LVSI
b. Up to stage I A1 with LVSI
c. Up to stage I A2 with no LVSI
d. Up to stage I A2 with LVSI

93. Percentage of lymphatic metastasis in microinvasive cancer cervix is:

a. <1%
b. <2%
c. <3%
d. <10%

94. True about SLN mapping in cancer cervix are all, *except*:

a. SLN detection rates 89–92%
b. Suspicious LNs need to be removed regardless of SLN mapping
c. Ipsilateral lymphadenectomy is omitted in case of failed SLN mapping
d. Best when tumor size is <2 cm diameter

95. True about involvement of the para-aortic LN in cancer cervix includes all, *except*:

a. Primary tumor size <2 cm
b. Primary tumor size >4 cm
c. Pelvic LN metastasis
d. Para-aortic lymph nodal dissection is recommended when ≥ stage I B1

96. SENTICOL study showed:

a. Limited agreement between lymphoscintigraphy and intraoperative SLN mapping
b. Bilateral SLN detection and biopsy is more reliable than unilateral SLN mapping
c. Included stage I A1 with LVSI to stage I B1
d. All of the above

97. As per the phase III Left Atrial Appendage Closure (LAAC) trial regarding the role of minimally invasive surgery (MIS) in cancer cervix is:

a. Mostly were stage I B1 disease
b. Lower rate of disease-free survival in MIS
c. Decrease in overall survival in MIS
d. All of the above

98. Recent evidences suggest that MIS in cancer cervix is associated with all, *except*:

a. Decrease in hospital stay
b. Decrease in morbidity
c. More rapid patient recovery
d. Increase in 5-year survival as compared to the open surgery

99. As per NCCN panel agreement:

a. Primary surgery for stage I A, I B1, I B2, and select II A1
b. Concurrent chemoradiation for stage I B3 to stage IV A
c. Concurrent chemoradiation for surgically unfit candidates
d. All of the above

100. Effective treatment can cure what percentage of stage I–II cancer cervix patients?

a. 40%
b. 50%
c. 60%
d. 80%

101. Effective treatment can cure what percentage of stage III cancer cervix patients?

a. 40%
b. 50%
c. 60%
d. 80%

102. Locally advanced disease cancer cervix is defined as:

a. Stage II B to stage IV A
b. Stage I B3 and stage II A2
c. Stage II A1 to stage IV B
d. Both a and b

103. As per NCCN; extra-fascial hysterectomy (type A) is ideally for:

a. Stage I A1
b. Stage I A1 with LVSI
c. Stage I A1 and stage I A2
d. Up to stage I B2

104. As per NCCN; modified radical hysterectomy (type B) is ideally for:

a. Stage I A1 with LVSI and stage I A2
b. Stage I A1
c. Up to stage I B1
d. Up to stage I B2

105. As per NCCN; radical hysterectomy (type C1) is ideally for:

a. Stage I B1 to stage I B2
b. Stage I A1 with LVSI and stage I A2
c. Selected stage I B3–II A1
d. Both a and c

106. As radical trachelectomy ideally for:

a. Stage I A2–I B1 and select I B2
b. Carcinoma in situ
c. Stage I A1
d. Stage II A1

107. As per NCCN guidelines MMR/MSI or PD-L1 ± NTRK gene fusion testing should be done for:

a. Recurrent disease
b. Progressive disease
c. Metastatic disease
d. All of the above

108. Drug of choice for PD-L1 or MSI-H/d MMR tumors is:

a. Pemetrexed
b. Vinorelbine
c. Bevacizumab
d. Pembrolizumab

109. False about ultrastaging of SLN means:

a. Serial sectioning of the gross LN
b. Review of H and E
c. With or without cytokeratin immunohistochemistry
d. All the above constitute standard protocol for ultrastaging SLN

110. True about trachelectomy includes all, *except*:

a. Mobilization in simple trachelectomy is up to peritoneal reflection
b. Mobilization in radical trachelectomy is up to upper vagina and below cervix
c. 5 mm of cranial part of cervix is left for cervical encirclage
d. Good oncologic outcome with minimally invasive trachelectomy is established

111. In posterior infralevator exenteration surgery with curative intent in select stage IV A cancer cervix unfit for radiotherapy:

a. Bladder and urethra preserved
b. Rectum is removed
c. Anal sphincter removed
d. All of the above

112. In anterior infralevator exenteration surgery with curative intent in select stage IV A cancer cervix unfit for radiotherapy:

a. Bladder and urethra removed
b. Rectum is preserved
c. Anal sphincter preserved
d. All of the above

113. In total infralevator exenteration surgery with curative intent in select stage IV A cancer cervix unfit for radiotherapy:

a. Bladder and urethra removed
b. Rectum removed
c. Anal sphincter removed
d. All of the above

114. In posterior supralevator exenteration surgery with curative intent in select stage IV A cancer cervix unfit for radiotherapy:

a. Bladder and urethra preserved
b. Rectum removed
c. Anal sphincter preserved
d. All of the above

115. In total supralevator exenteration surgery with curative intent in select stage IV A cancer cervix unfit for radiotherapy:

a. Bladder and urethra removed
b. Rectum removed
c. Anal sphincter preserved
d. All of the above

116. Good prognostic type A endocervical adenocarcinomas include all, *except*:

a. Well-demarcated glands with round contours
b. Absence of desmoplastic stromal response
c. Presence of single cells
d. Absence of LVSI

117. What is the increase in the incidence of benign ovarian cysts after an ovarian transposition surgery?

a. Twofold increase
b. Threefold increase
c. Fourfold increase
d. No increase in incidence

118. Gynecologic Oncology Group score for cervical cancer recurrence includes all, *except*:

a. Clinical size of the tumor
b. Parametrial extension
c. Presence or absence of LVSI
d. Depth of stromal invasion

119. Tumor markers used in cancer cervix include all, *except*:

a. CA125
b. Serum squamous cell carcinoma antigen
c. HPV type
d. Epidermal growth factor receptor

120. Positive peritoneal cytology is an independent prognostic factor in which type of cancer cervix?

a. Adenocarcinoma
b. Adenosquamous
c. Small cell neuroendocrine carcinoma
d. None of the above

121. Percentage of adenocarcinoma amongst invasive cervical cancer is:

a. 5%
b. 10%
c. 15%
d. 30%

122. Human papillomavirus with greater propensity of persistence:

a. HPV16
b. HPV18
c. HPV31
d. HPV33

123. Increased risk of the adenocarcinoma variant of cervical cancer includes all, *except*:

a. Obesity
b. Smoking
c. Oral contraceptives
d. HPV16 and HPV18

ANSWERS KEY

1. d	2. b	3. d	4. d	5. d	6. a	7. c
8. b	9. b	10. c	11. a	12. c	13. a	14. c
15. a	16. a	17. a	18. c	19. c	20. d	21. a
22. b	23. b	24. a	25. c	26. c	27. b	28. b
29. b	30. a	31. a	32. c	33. a	34. a	35. d
36. a	37. d	38. a	39. c	40. d	41. d	42. c
43. b	44. d	45. a	46. c	47. c	48. d	49. a
50. d	51. d	52. b	53. d	54. c	55. d	56. d
57. a	58. a	59. d	60. d	61. d	62. d	63. d
64. a	65. a	66. a	67. a	68. d	69. d	70. d
71. d	72. d	73. b	74. d	75. a	76. d	77. a
78. b	79. b	80. c	81. d	82. d	83. d	84. b
85. d	86. b	87. d	88. a	89. a	90. d	91. d

Contd...

Contd...

92. a	93. a	94. c	95. a	96. d	97. d	98. d
99. d	100. d	101. c	102. d	103. a	104. a	105. d
106. a	107. d	108. d	109. d	110. d	111. d	112. d
113. d	114. d	115. d	116. c	117. b	118. b	119. a
120. a	121. c	122. a	123. b			

NOTES: CERVICAL CANCER

- Prof Dr Neerja Bhatla, AIIMS (New Delhi), and team have been instrumental in making the revised new FIGO staging of cancer cervix (2018). This is a landmark contribution and perhaps the greatest by any Indian so far.
- The changes in the new staging are:
    - The lateral extent of the disease has been removed from stage I A
    - Presence of LVSI do not affect the stage of the disease
    - Stage I B has got three subgroups
    - Radiology (r) or pathology (p) can be used to determine the size of the lesion
    - Radiology (TVS/CT/MRI/PET) or pathology can be used to assess the status of the retroperitoneal LNs
    - When in doubt regarding the correct stage, lower stage should be assigned
    - Isolated tumor cells do not change the stage but their presence should be noted.
- Cervical cancer is more common in women who have not had any regular screening (Pap smear or HPV DNA testing).
- Also, diagnosis is often delayed in those who have had not undergone any regular screening.
- Postcoital bleeding is a classical symptom. Cervical cancer is in fact a late advanced staged presentation in those who are not sexually active.
- In absence of any obvious cervical growth but unusually firm of expanded should undergo a biopsy and an endocervical curettage.
- Lymph nodes >1 cm is usually considered positive in CT scan.
- Magnetic resonance imaging accuracy in cervical cancer, as per the revised latest edition of standard books:

- Tumor size (93%)
- Depth of stromal invasion (78%)
- Parametrial invasion (94%) and it is 76% in CT scan
- Uterine body involvement is associated with the risk of LN involvement.
- Lymph nodal spread in cervical cancer goes from the pelvic sidewall nodes to the common iliac nodes and then to the para-aortic LNs. However, unexpected places like presacral nodes may also get involved and this zone is actually not addressed in case of a radical hysterectomy (*see* the lymphatic routes of cervix by Reiffenstuhl in Te Linde's operative gynecology).
- Microinvasive cervical cancer means depth of invasion up to 5 mm and that LVSI is absent (stage I A1 and stage 1 A2).
- There is appositive corelation between the depth of invasion and LVSI but it says that there is no positive corelation between LVSI and that of lymph nodal involvement.
- Fertility preserving surgery can be offered to stage I A2 but the recommended treatment for stage 1 A2 is modified radical hysterectomy with pelvic LN dissection. Again, fertility sparing radical trachelectomy with pelvic LN dissection can be extended up to stage I B1 cases. All authorities agree that fertility sparing surgery can be offered to lesion size ≤2 cm.
- The adenocarcinoma variant can be multifocal in origin unlike that of squamous counterpart.
- Equal cure rates are seen with both primary radiation therapy and radical hysterectomy with pelvic LN dissection for stage I B1 and stage I B2.
- Chronological age should not be considered a contraindication to radical surgery. Morbidity of surgery is found to be same for both.
- Type I extra-fascial hysterectomy—Stage I A1.
- Type II modified radical hysterectomy—Stage I A2.
- Type III radical hysterectomy—Stage I B up to stage II A2.
- Kyoto classification of hysterectomies (Querleu and Morrow): Lateral extent of the disease.

Type A	Minimum resection of the paracervix and vaginal resection <10 mm (similar to type I as above)
Type B	Transection of paracervix at the ureter (similar to type II) B1—without removal of lateral paracervical LNs B2—with removal of the lateral paracervical LNs
Type C	Transection of the paracervix at the junction with the internal iliac vascular system (similar to type III) C1—with nerve preservation. The uterosacral is transected afterseparation of the hypogastric nerves C2—without preservation of autonomic nerves. The paracervix is transected completely including the part caudal to the deep uterine vein
Type D	Laterally extended resections D1—resection of the entire paracervix at the pelvic sidewall, along withthe hypogastric and obturator vessels, exposing the roots of the sciatic nerve D2—resection of the entire paracervix along with the hypogastric vessels and adjacent fascial or muscular components

- Lymph node dissection levels:

Level 1: External and internal iliac
Level 2: Common iliac (it includes presacral LN)
Level 3: Aortic inframesenteric
Level 4: Aortic infrarenal

- New thought process in pelvic lymphadenectomy:
  - In case of bulky and frozen section positive pelvic or para-aortic LN: Only enlarged LNs are to be removed and CCRT will control the micrometastasis.
  - It is proposed that a thorough lymphadenectomy is of therapeutic value for nodes negative early cervical cancer
  - *In the presence of positive LNs*: Preferred is to proceed with the radical hysterectomy as it removes the primary lesion and avoids the need for brachytherapy. Disease free survival rate is better and there is significantly lower chance of pelvic recurrences but the overall survival is not so different.
- Sentinel lymph node mapping and ultrastaging in early cervical cancer presently has got a false-negative rate of 1.3% in best of the centers.
- Urodynamic morbidity is significantly reduced with nerve sparing radical hysterectomy. Although, nerve sparing radical hysterectomy is more of a conservative type of radical hysterectomy; there is no increase in recurrence rate when compared with the classical radical hysterectomy.
- Postoperative complications of radical hysterectomy:
  - Prolonged ileus may be due to lymphatic ascites.
  - Hypertonic bladder with elevated urethral pressure is the most common bladder dysfunction.
  - Hypotonic bladder complication is the worst prognostic one.
  - Sexual dysfunction can be in 55% cases.
  - Lymphedema can be seen in 20% cases. It is increased whenever radiotherapy is added after the surgery.
- Prognostic marker for early-staged cancer cervix:
  - Status of LNs (most important prognostic marker)
  - Size of primary tumor
  - Depth of stromal invasion
  - Presence or absence of LVSI
  - Presence or absence of parametrial extension
  - Histologic cell type
  - Status of vaginal margins
  - Treatment in a high-volume center
  - Tumor marker
  - Microvessel density
  - Morbid obesity

- Prognostic GOG score > 120 indicates a possible recurrence of 40% at 3 years.
- 5-year survival with parametrial invasion is about 62%.
- Close vaginal margin is when the cut margin has a distance of ≤5 mm.
- High levels of ribonucleotide reductase (RNR) inhibitors are associated with a worse prognosis and can be monitored during the treatment of CCRT.
- Immunotherapy used in cancer cervix includes axalimogene filolisbac (live irreversibly attenuated *Listeria monocytogenes*) and pembrolizumab (immune checkpoint inhibitors).
- KEYNOTE trials for use of Pembrolizumab.
- *New radiation modalities*: Image guided brachytherapy, Intensity modulated radiation therapy (IMRT), Volumetric modulated arc therapy (VMAT) and Intraoperative radiotherapy (IORT).
- *NACT in cancer cervix*: Prague study offered to Stage I B 2 (Both squamous and adenocarcinoma types) and there was radical hysterectomy in 94% cases and post-operative radiation in 26.7% patients. 5-year disease specific survival was noted to be 83.6% (median follow-up time period of 88.5 months).
  NACT is a treatment of choice in case of cancer cervix in pregnancy who wish to continue her pregnancy and is followed by Radical Cesarean Hysterectomy.
- *Pelvic exenteration*: Most common indication is central recurrence or persistent central disease after radiation therapy in Cancer Cervix. Pre-operative PET-CT and diagnostic laparoscopy is helpful in the assessing the disease extent.
- Anterior exenteration involves removal of uterus, cervix, bladder, urethra and anterior vagina, at times along with vulva while posterior vagina and rectum are preserved. Posterior exenteration involves removal of rectum and posterior vagina (but many surgeons do removal of distal ureter, urinary bladder and urethra to avoid post-operative urinary fistula and thus converting them into total exenteration).
- Total pelvic exenteration is the most common approach for central recurrence in cancer cervix. Total exenteration can be supra-levator or it can include levator muscle also. Mortality rate is 5% and around 50% may have major complications (fistula, bowel obstruction and pyelonephritis). Pre-operative counseling including psycho-social rehabilitation is very important to understand the balance between expectations and outcome. Negative prognostic indicators of pelvic exenteration are central recurrence greater than 3 cm, lymphatic spread, parametrial involvement and disease-free interval of less than 1 year. Side-wall involvement or hydronephrosis or nodal involvement are contraindications for pelvic exenteration.

- Minimally Invasive versus Abdominal Radical Hysterectomy for Cervical Cancer by Pedro T. Ramirez et al. In this trial, minimally invasive radical hysterectomy was associated with lower rates of disease-free survival and overall survival than open abdominal radical hysterectomy among women with early-stage cervical cancer. (November 15, 2018 N Engl J Med. 2018; 379:1895-1904 DOI: 10.1056/NEJMoa1806395)
- Survival After Minimally Invasive vs Open Radical Hysterectomy for Early-Stage Cervical Cancer: A Systematic Review and Meta-analysis. Roni Nitecki et al. This systematic review and meta-analysis of observational studies found that among patients undergoing radical hysterectomy for early-stage cervical cancer, minimally invasive radical hysterectomy was associated with an elevated risk of recurrence and death compared with open surgery. (JAMA Oncol. 2020;6(7):1019-1027. doi:10.1001/jamaoncol.2020.1694 Published online June 11, 2020).

Uterine Cancer and Other Uterine Malignancies

1. Nonendometrioid endometrial cancer mutations include:

a. PTEN

b. β-catenin

c. p53

d. K-ras

2. Endometrioid endometrial cancer mutations include all, *except*:

a. PTEN

b. β-catenin

c. p53

d. K-ras

3. Type II endometrial cancer risk factors includes all, *except*:

a. Older women

b. Obese women

c. Multiparous

d. Tamoxifen

4. Type I endometrial cancer risk factors includes all, *except*:

a. 5-year survival rate of approximately 83%

b. Obese women

c. Mean age of onset is 70 years

d. Current smokers

5. What percentage of women with endometrial cancer has malignant cells on Pap smear?

a. 20%

b. 30%

c. 40%

d. 50%

6. What percentage of women with abnormal endometrial cells in Pap smear will have endometrial carcinoma?

a. 20%

b. 25%

c. 30%

d. 35%

7. Detection rate of endometrial cancer by pipelle in postmenopausal women is:

a. 71%

b. 81%

c. 91%

d. 99.6%

8. Detection rate of endometrial cancer by pipelle in premenopausal women is:

a. 71%

b. 91%

c. 81%

d. 61%

9. False negative rate of transvaginal ultrasonography for endometrial cancer is:

a. 4%
b. 8%
c. 40%
d. 50%

10. False positive rate of transvaginal ultrasonography for endometrial cancer is:

a. 4%
b. 8%
c. 40%
d. 50%

11. Tamoxifen increases the risk of endometrial cancer by:

a. Twofolds
b. 2–3 folds
c. 3–4 folds
d. 4–5 folds

12. Most common cause of postmenopausal bleeding is:

a. Endometrial hyperplasia
b. Exogenous estrogens
c. Atrophic endometritis/vaginitis
d. Endometrial cancers

13. Postmenopausal bleeding due to endometrial cancer accounts to:

a. 5%
b. 10%
c. 15%
d. 20%

14. False negative rate of endometrial biopsy for endometrial cancer is:

a. 2%
b. 5%
c. 10%
d. 15%

15. Accuracy of myometrial invasion by magnetic resonance imaging (MRI) in endometrial cancer is:

a. 73%
b. 83%
c. 93%
d. 95%

16. Positive predictive value of MRI for cervical involvement in endometrial cancer is:

a. 100%
b. 90%
c. 80%
d. 70%

17. What is the percentage of nonsquamous solid growth pattern in grade 2 endometrial cancer?

a. 5%
b. 6–60%
c. 6–50%
d. 6–40%

18. Screening for genetic mutations in endometrial cancer should be done in all:

a. Endometrial cancer in <50 years age
b. Significant family history of colorectal cancer

   c. Significant family history of endometrial cancer

   d. All of the above

19. **Validated screening test for endometrial cancer:**

   a. CA125

   b. Transvaginal ultrasound

   c. Pap smear

   d. None of the above

20. **As per International Federation of Gynecology and Obstetrics (FIGO) 2009 staging; endometrial cancer involving the vagina:**

   a. Stage III A

   b. Stage III B

   c. Stage III C

   d. Stage IV B

21. **As per FIGO 2009, endometrial cancer involving the serosa of the uterus or adnexa:**

   a. Stage III A

   b. Stage III B

   c. Stage III C

   d. Stage IV B

22. **Endometrial cancer involving the parametrium as per FIGO staging 2009:**

   a. Stage III A

   b. Stage III B

   c. Stage III C

   d. Stage IV B

23. **Endometrial cancers involving the pelvic nodes as per FIGO staging 2009:**

   a. Staging III A

   b. Staging III B

   c. Staging III C1

   d. Staging III C2

24. **Endometrial cancers involving inguinal lymph nodal metastasis as per FIGO staging 2009:**

   a. Stage IV A

   b. Stage IV B

   c. Stage III C

   d. Stage III B

25. **Endometrial cancers involving omental metastasis as per FIGO staging 2009:**

   a. Stage IV A

   b. Stage IV B

   c. Stage III C

   d. Stage III B

26. **Most common mode of spread in endometrial cancer is:**

   a. Hematogenous

   b. Lymphatics

   c. Transtubal

   d. Direct extension

27. **Predictor of vaginal recurrences in endometrial cancer includes all, *except*:**

   a. Grade 3

   b. LVSI

   c. Depth of myometrial invasion

   d. Stage of the lesion

28. **Predictor of distant metastasis in cancer endometrium includes:**

    a. Grade   b. Myometrial invasion
    c. LVSI   d. All of the above

29. **Low risk for lymph node metastasis includes all, except:**

    a. Tumor size <2 cm
    b. <50% myometrial invasion
    c. Well-differentiated or moderately-differentiated histology
    d. Presence of lower uterine segment involvement

(Positive cytology along with the presence of other adverse risk factors is a risk factor for lymph nodal metastasis)

30. **Percentage of lymph node metastasis with tumor size >2 cm in endometrial cancer is:**

    a. 4%   b. 15%
    c. 25%   d. 35%

31. **Not an independent prognostic factor in endometrial cancer is:**

    a. Peritoneal cytology   b. Histologic grade
    c. Myometrial invasion   d. LVSI

32. **True about coexistent cancer endometrium and complex atypical endometrial hyperplasia includes:**

    a. 48% on hysterectomy specimen
    b. 30% on D and C specimen
    c. Increased prediction with cotesting for PTEN, MIB-I, and p53
    d. All of the above

33. **Surgical staging in endometrial cancers depends upon:**

    a. Grade   b. Myometrial invasion
    c. Histology   d. Size of the lesion
    e. All of the above

34. **Percentage of negative para-aortic nodes when the pelvic nodes are negative:**

    a. 66%   b. 76%
    c. 86%   d. 96%

35. **Percentage of positive para-aortic nodes when the pelvic lymph nodes are positive:**

    a. 28%   b. 30%
    c. 35%   d. 48%

36. **Best method to perform sentinel lymph node (SLN) biopsy in endometrial cancer:**

    a. Cervical injection   b. Hysteroscopic technique
    c. Subserosal injection technique   d. None of the above

(Cervical injection with indigo cyanine green dye is one of the best options. Other options include combined use of blue dye and radioactive tracer).

37. As per PORTEC-2 (Postoperative Radiation Therapy in Endometrial Carcinoma) study, vaginal recurrences after brachytherapy in high-intermediate risk diseases are:
   a. 1.8%
   b. 2.8%
   c. 3.8%
   d. 1.6%

38. As per PORTEC-2 study, vaginal recurrences after external beam therapy in high-intermediate risk diseases are:
   a. 1.8%
   b. 2.8%
   c. 3.8%
   d. 1.6%

39. Synchronous ovarian epithelial cancer and endometrial cancers occur in:
   a. 3–5%
   b. 5–10%
   c. 10–15%
   d. 15–20%

40. Endometrial cancer is the sentinel cancer for Lynch syndrome in about:
   a. 25%
   b. 50%
   c. 75%
   d. 10%

41. Approximately, what percentage of recurrences occurs beyond 5 years of treatment in endometrial cancers?
   a. 10%
   b. 15%
   c. 20%
   d. 5%

42. Risk factors for uterine sarcoma include all, *except*:
   a. Pelvic radiation
   b. HRT ≥ 5 years
   c. OCP ≥ 5 years
   d. Myomas with chromosomal 2 defect

43. Malignant mixed mesodermal tumors (MMMT) present with enlarged uterus and protrudes as polyp through os in:
   a. 60%
   b. 50%
   c. 40%
   d. 30%

44. What percentage of carcinosarcomas has prior history of pelvic radiation?
   a. 17%
   b. 27%
   c. 37%
   d. 47%

45. Myoma with which chromosomal number defects gives rise to sarcoma?

a. Chromosome 1

b. Chromosome 2

c. Chromosome 3

d. Chromosome 4

46. Radiation therapy when indicated after surgical staging in endometrial cancer should not be initiated later than:

a. 6 weeks after surgery

b. 8 weeks after surgery

c. 10 weeks after surgery

d. 12 weeks after surgery

47. High-risk factors in cancer endometrium include:

a. Age

b. LVSI

c. Depth of myometrial invasion

d. All of the above

48. Use of CA 125 in cancer endometrium corelates includes all, *except*:

a. Marker of extrauterine spread

b. Grade of tumor

c. Prognostic marker

d. No role in deciding adjuvant treatment

49. True about fertility sparing surgery in endometrial cancer includes all, *except*:

a. Well-differentiated endometrioid adenocarcinoma

b. Disease limited to the uterus

c. No contraindications to medical therapy

d. Standard of care

50. Staging in endometrial cancer is not affected by:

a. Depth of myometrial invasion

b. Cytology of peritoneal fluid

c. Tumor size

d. Level of nodal involvement

51. Ultrastaging of SLN includes:

a. Serial sectioning with H and E staining

b. Review of slides

c. Cytokeratin IHC staining

d. All of the above

52. Preferred chemotherapeutic regimens for HER2-positive uterine serous carcinoma is:

a. Carboplatin

b. Paclitaxel

c. Trastuzumab

d. All of the above

53. Preferred chemotherapeutic agents for uterine sarcoma include all, *except*:

a. Doxorubicin
b. Docetaxel
c. Gemcitabine
d. Ifosfamide

54. Preferred chemotherapeutic agents for low-grade endometrial stromal sarcoma are:

a. Aromatase inhibitors
b. GnRH analogues
c. Megestrol acetate
d. Medroxyprogesterone acetate

55. Designation used when tumor grade cannot be assessed is:

a. GX
b. G0
c. Gx
d. GA

56. FIRES trial includes:

a. Comparison between SLN mapping and complete lymphadenectomy
b. SLN was successful in 86% of the patients
c. Sensitivity of 97.2%
d. All of the above

57. Sentinel lymph node ultrastaging can lead to upstaging of disease in:

a. 2–5%
b. 5–15%
c. 15–25%
d. 20–40%

58. Recent studies approve SLN in all, *except*:

a. Clear cell adenocarcinoma
b. Serous adenocarcinoma
c. Carcinosarcoma
d. Uterine Sarcoma

59. Gynecologic Oncology Group (GOG)-LAP 2 trial (laparoscopic surgical staging in endometrial cancer) include all, *except*:

a. 26% conversion of MIS into open laparotomy
b. Overall survival 84.8% in both arms
c. Lymph node removal was more in laparoscopy arm
d. 11.4% recurrence in laparoscopy and 10.2% recurrence in laparotomy arm

60. Laparoscopic Approach to Cancer of the Endometrium (LACE) trial:

a. No difference in overall survival and recurrence in both arms
b. Stage I endometrial cancer
c. Compared open versus laparoscopic hysterectomy
d. All of the above

61. Best modality to differentiate uterine leiomyosarcomas from degenerating leiomyomas is:

a. Total serum LDH
b. MRI
c. Dynamic MRI
d. LDH and dynamic MRI

62. **Increased relative risk of uterine cancer is associated with all, *except*:**

a. Use of oral contraceptives
b. Late-onset menopause
c. Early-onset menarche
d. Nulliparity

63. **Decreased relative risk of uterine cancer is associated with all, *except*:**

a. Use of oral contraceptives
b. Cigarette smoking
c. Infertility
d. Physical activity

64. **Minimum duration of progesterone in a month to be given for risk reduction of uterine cancer:**

a. 10 days
b. 12 days
c. 16 days
d. 28 days

65. **Over all 5-year survival rate of low grade endometrial stromal sarcomas:**

a. 90.1%
b. 70.1%
c. 50.6%
d. 32.6%

66. **Age-adjusted mortality rate of endometrial cancer per 100,000 women is:**

a. 3.5
b. 4.5
c. 5.5
d. 7.5

67. **Overall 5-year survival rate of endometrial cancer is:**

a. 40.8%
b. 60.5%
c. 83.8%
d. 90.4%

68. **High risk of lymph node involvement in endometrial cancer includes all *except*:**

a. Tumor size > 2 cm
b. Only positive cytology for malignant cells
c. Positive LVSI
d. Deep myometrial invasion

69. **Relative risk of endometrial cancer in presence of obesity:**

a. 1.5
b. 2.5
c. 3.5
d. 4.5

70. **Over all 5-year survival rate of high grade endometrial stromal sarcoma:**

a. 82%
b. 62%
c. 52%
d. 32%

ANSWERS KEY

1. c	2. c	3. b	4. c	5. d	6. b	7. d
8. b	9. a	10. d	11. b	12. c	13. c	14. c
15. b	16. b	17. c	18. d	19. d	20. b	21. a
22. b	23. c	24. b	25. b	26. d	27. c	28. d
29. d	30. b	31. a	32. d	33. e	34. d	35. d
36. d	37. a	38. d	39. a	40. b	41. a	42. d
43. b	44. c	45. a	46. d	47. d	48. d	49. d
50. b	51. d	52. d	53. d	54. a	55. a	56. d
57. b	58. d	59. c	60. d	61. d	62. a	63. c
64. a	65. a	66. b	67. c	68. b	69 b	70. d

NOTES: ENDOMETRIAL CANCER

- *Molecular classification of endometrial cancer (Cancer Genome Atlas Project):*
  - *Group 1 (7%):* Ultramutated group with POLE DNA polymerase mutation. Associated with good prognosis
  - *Group 2 (28%):* Hypermutated group with microsatellite instability and defects in mismatch repair.
  - *Group 3 (39%):* Low-copy number group that exhibited microsatellite instability.
  - *Group 4 (26%):* Characterized by a low mutation group, chromosomal instability, and high copy number variations. Mostly with TP53 mutations, grade 3 tumor, and serous carcinomas. It is associated with worst prognosis.
- Recent meta-analysis is suggesting that 3 mm should be the cut-off of endometrial thickness for investigations in to a case of postmenopausal bleeding.
- Most common mode of spread in endometrial cancer is direct spread.
- Etiologies of postmenopausal bleeding are:
  - Exogenous estrogens (30%)
  - Atrophic endometritis/vaginitis (30%)

- Endometrial cancer (15%)
- Endometrial or cervical polyps (10%)
- Endometrial hyperplasia (5%)
- Miscellaneous (cervical cancer, uterine sarcoma, urethral caruncle, and trauma) (10%)
- *High suspicion of endometrial cancer:*
  - All patients with postmenopausal bleeding
  - Postmenopausal women with pyometra
  - Asymptomatic postmenopausal women with endometrial cells on pap smear
  - Abnormal menstrual bleeding in perimenopausal women
- Endometrial hyperplasia is used for any degree of glandular proliferation devoid of cytologic atypia and endometrial intraepithelial neoplasia (EIN) for lesions with cytologic atypia. Biologically, these two are two different diseases.
- *World Health Organization (WHO) classification of endometrial cancer:*
  - *Hyperplasia (1–3% risk of developing endometrial cancer):* Simple hyperplasia without atypia and complex hyperplasia without atypia
  - *Atypical hyperplasia (8–28% risk of developing endometrial cancer):* Simple atypical hyperplasia and complex atypical hyperplasia
- *Prognostic variables in endometrial cancer are:*
  - Stage of the disease
  - Age
  - Histologic type and grade
  - Nuclear grade
  - Myometrial invasion
  - Lymphovascular space invasion (LVSI)
  - Tumor size
  - Peritoneal cytology
  - Hormone receptor status
  - DNA ploidy and other biologic markers
  - Body mass index
  - Type of therapy (Surgery Vs Radiotherapy)
- Age below 40 years has good prognostic outcome.
- *Poor prognostic factor in terms of histological patterns:* Serous carcinomas, clear cell carcinomas, and squamous cell carcinomas.
- *In case of mixed serous and endometrioid patterns:* Poor prognosis when serous component >25%.
- *Grade 1 lesions and inner one-third myometrial invasion:* 3% positive pelvic nodes.
- *Grade 3 lesions and outer one-third myometrial invasion:* 34% positive pelvic nodes.
- Vascular space invasion carries a risk of death of 1.5 times.

- LVSI is an independent risk factor for vaginal cuff recurrence, distant metastasis, lymph node metastasis, parametrial invasion even in early-staged endometrial cancer. Substantial LVSI is associated with locoregional recurrence, distant metastasis, and overall survival.
- Positive peritoneal cytology is no longer an independent prognostic marker and rather it reflects the presence of other adverse factors. But, positive peritoneal cytology in absence of other risk factors does not carry any prognostic significance.
- Presence of estrogen receptor (ER) and progesterone receptor (PR) carries good prognosis. PR appears to be stronger predictor of survival than ER receptor.
- Nuclear grade is more accurate prognostic marker than the histological grade.
- Tumor size > 2 cm and lower uterine segment involvement is associated with positive pelvic lymph nodes.
- 25% of endometrial cancer carry aneuploid tumors. Aneuploid tumors have increased risk of early recurrence and carries a 4.1 relative risk of death.
- BMI ≥ 40 carries poor outcome.
- If pelvic nodes are positive, then 50% of patients will have positive para-aortic nodes. But when pelvic nodes are negative; only about 2% of patients will have isolated para-aortic metastasis.
- *Potential roles of lymphadenectomy*:
  - Surgical staging
  - Positive nodes are eliminated (no preoperative method can detect micrometastasis in lymph nodes)
  - Directs adjuvant treatment
  - Extensive para-aortic lymph nodes can be avoided in elderly morbidly obsese patients as it can entail higher postoperative morbidity in this subgroup of patients.
- *Further study*: ASTEC (A Study in the Treatment of Endometrial Cancer) to assess the efficacy of pelvic lymphadenectomy in endometrial cancer.
- *PORTEC 1*: Surgery (TAH + BSO without pelvic lymphadenectomy) and postoperative external pelvic radiation versus surgery alone:
  - Postoperative radiation therapy was not indicated in patients with stage I endometrial cancer < 60 years of age and in patients with grade 2 tumors with superficial invasion.
  - Radiotherapy was indicated for high-risk patients who were not staged surgically as it gives locoregional benefits.
- *PORTEC 2*: Whether vaginal brachytherapy was effective as pelvic external-beam radiation for patients with high-intermediate risk disease.
  - Vaginal brachytherapy is associated with lower side-effects but with higher pelvic recurrences.

- But, there were no differences in overall or disease-free survival in the groups.
- *PORTEC 3*: Adjuvant chemoradiotherapy (CRT) versus radiotherapy (RT) alone following surgery.
  - 5-year failure free survival for stage I–II patients was 80.8% in the CRT group compared to 68.6% with RT alone. Patients with stage III disease had an 11% absolute improvement of failure-free survival with CRT. CRT is associated with more adverse side-effects.
- LACE Trial (Laparoscopic Approach to Cancer of the Endometrium): Validates the use of laparoscopic approach in early staged cancer endometrium (Stage I).
- Treatment of choice for stage II endometrial cancer is type II radical hysterectomy plus bilateral salpingo-oophorectomy and lymphadenectomy (pelvic and para-aortic), omental biopsy, excision of any pelvic or abdominal nodules, and peritoneal wash cytology followed by individualized adjuvant radiation.
- Endometrial carcinoma in young patients is usually found in case of infertility patients with polycystic ovarian syndrome.
- Symptomatic patients post-treatment of endometrial cancer can be offered hormone replacement therapy (studies conferred no increase in recurrence with the use of HRT). Conjugated estrogen or tibolone may be used.
- *Uterine Smooth Muscle Tumor of Uncertain Malignant Potential (STUMP)*: Poor understood clinical behavior.
- WHO classifies endometrial stromal tumors into four categories:
  1. Benign endometrial nodules
  2. Low-grade endometrial stromal sarcomas
  3. High-grade endometrial stromal sarcomas
  4. Undifferentiated uterine sarcomas
- Malignant mixed mesodermal tumors or carcinosarcomas usually occur in older age group. They are surgically staged same as carcinomas.

Epithelial Ovarian Cancer

1. Woman's risk at birth of having ovarian cancer in her lifetime is:

a. 1%

b. 2%

c. 3%

d. 4%

2. True about type II high-grade ovarian cancers includes all, *except*:

a. Originates from the mucosa of fallopian tube

b. Involves p53 mutations

c. Develops slowly

d. Presents at advanced stage

3. Percentage of ovarian neoplasms being malignant in premenopausal women is:

a. 7%

b. 10%

c. 20%

d. 30%

4. Percentage of ovarian neoplasms being malignant in postmenopausal women is:

a. 7%

b. 10%

c. 20%

d. 30%

5. Risk of ovarian malignancy includes all, *except*:

a. Childhood obesity and high body mass index (BMI)

b. Infertility

c. Nulliparity

d. Infertility drugs

6. 5 years or more use of oral contraceptive pills (OCPs) causes an ovarian cancer risk reduction of what percentage?

a. 20%

b. 30%

c. 50%

d. 70%

7. A woman with two children and have used OCPs for 5 years or more causes a ovarian cancer risk reduction by:

a. 20%

b. 30%

c. 50%

d. 70%

8. **Risk reducing prophylactic surgery in women with *BRCA-1* and *BRCA-2* mutations includes:**

a. Removal of both ovaries only
b. Removal of both ovaries and both fallopian tubes only
c. Removal of both fallopian tubes only
d. Removal of both ovaries, both fallopian tubes, and total peritonectomy

9. **Cost-effective method of reducing risk of ovarian cancer in *BRCA* mutations women:**

a. Risk reducing bilateral salpingo-oophorectomy
b. Annual pelvic examinations
c. Annual CA125 and transvaginal ultrasound
d. All of the above

10. **Fertility preservation surgery in epithelial ovarian cancer is an option in all, *except*:**

a. Stage I A (grade I and grade II) serous or mucinous or endometrioid types
b. Stage I C (grade I and grade II) serous or mucinous or endometrioid types
c. Stage I A clear cell carcinoma
d. Stage I A and stage I C (grade III) and stage I C clear cell carcinoma

11. **Percentage of ovarian cancer due to germ-line mutations in *BRCA-1* and *BRCA-2* is:**

a. 5–10%
b. 10–14%
c. 15–20%
d. 21–25%

12. ***BRCA-1* gene is located in:**

a. Chromosome 17
b. Chromosome 13
c. Chromosome 11
d. Chromosome 18

13. ***BRCA-2* gene is located in:**

a. Chromosome 17
b. Chromosome 13
c. Chromosome 11
d. Chromosome 18

14. **Family history is absent in what percentage of mutation positive ovarian cancers?**

a. 20%
b. 30%
c. 44%
d. 54%

15. "Founder effect" means higher rate of mutations have occurred within a specific:
- a. Period of time
- b. Population within a specific time
- c. Defined geographical areas within a specific time
- d. Population within a defined geographical area

16. The carrier rate of mutations in Ashkenazi Jewish for ovarian cancer is:
- a. 1.5%
- b. 2.5%
- c. 3.5%
- d. 7.5%

17. Prophylactic salpingo-oophorectomy reduces the risk of *BRCA*-related gynecologic cancer by:
- a. 96%
- b. 86%
- c. 76%
- d. 66%

18. Prophylactic salpingo-oophorectomy in premenopausal women reduces the risk of breast cancer by:
- a. 50–80%
- b. 60–90%
- c. 30–40%
- d. 20–30%

19. A *BRCA*-mutated patient who had undergone prophylactic salpingo-oophorectomy still carries a risk of primary peritoneal carcinoma of:
- a. 2–3%
- b. 4–5%
- c. 0.8–1%
- d. 0.3–0.5%

20. Hydrops tubae profluens associated with fallopian tube cancer is found in:
- a. ≤50%
- b. ≤30%
- c. ≤25%
- d. ≤15%

21. Hydrops tubae profluens associated with fallopian tube cancer includes all, *except*:
- a. Watery vaginal discharge
- b. Bleeding per vaginum
- c. Pelvic pain
- d. Pelvic mass

22. Most common mode of spread in malignant ovarian tumor is by:
- a. Transcoelomic
- b. Lymphatic
- c. Hematogenous
- d. Direct spread

23. Independent prognostic variables in ovarian malignancy include all, *except*:
- a. Patient's age
- b. Performance status
- c. Volume of ascites
- d. Histological grade

24. Overall survival of ovarian cancer patient in stage I is:

a. 20%
b. 30%
c. 60%
d. 80%

25. In ovarian malignancy, intraoperative surgical spill is considered to be:

a. Stage I C1
b. Stage I C2
c. Stage I C3
d. Stage II

26. In ovarian malignancy, pleural effusion with positive cytology is assigned as:

a. Stage III B
b. Stage III C
c. Stage IV A
d. Stage IV B

27. Omental deposits of ≥2 cm without positive retroperitoneal lymph nodes in ovarian malignancy is:

a. Stage III B
b. Stage III C
c. Stage IV A
d. Stage IV B

28. True in ovarian cancer prognosis includes all, *except*:

a. Histologic grade as predictor of occult metastasis
b. Positive cytology in early-staged disease
c. Capsular rupture in early-staged disease
d. Dense adhesions have got no prognostic value

29. Recurrence rate after a fertility sparing surgery in borderline ovarian tumor is:

a. 18.5%
b. 28.5%
c. 8.5%
d. 38.5%

30. Accuracy of the computed tomography (CT) scan in predicting suboptimal cytoreduction is:

a. 24%
b. 34%
c. 44%
d. 54%

(*Note:* In some studies, PPV of CT scan ~68%)

31. All are true about cytoreductive surgery, *except*:

a. Improves the nutritional status by enhancing physiology
b. Improves tumor perfusion
c. Decreases the chances of resistant clones of malignant cells
d. All of the above

32. Systemic pelvic and para-aortic lymphadenectomy in an optimally-cytoreduced patient includes all, *except*:

a. 6 month improvement in PFS
b. Overall 5-year survival increases

  c. No advantage seen if any macroscopic residual disease is left
  d. No increase in overall 5-year survival status

33. **Strongest predictor of overall survival in ovarian cancer is:**
  a. Performance status
  b. CA125
  c. Stage of the disease
  d. Complete tumor resection in either primary cytoreduction or interval cytoreduction

34. **In an optimally surgically cytoreduced early ovarian cancer; adjuvant chemotherapy is not required for the following, *except*:**
  a. Stage I grade 1
  b. Stage I grade 2
  c. Stage I grade 3
  d. Stage II grade 1 and 2

35. **Granulocyte colony-stimulating factors (G-CSF) is used for prevention and treatment of:**
  a. Neutropenia
  b. Neurotoxicity
  c. Nephrotoxicity
  d. All of the above

36. **Conventionally, platinum sensitive ovarian cancer means:**
  a. Relapsed free state for at least 03 months
  b. Relapsed free state for at least 06 months
  c. Relapsed free state for at least 09 months
  d. Relapsed free state for at least 12 months

37. **Platinum-resistant ovarian cancer means:**
  a. Disease progression within 3 months of completion of chemotherapy
  b. Disease progression within 6 months of completion of chemotherapy
  c. Disease progression within 9 months of completion of chemotherapy
  d. Disease progression within 12 months of completion of chemotherapy

38. **Hand-foot syndrome or acral erythema (palmar-plantar erythrodysesthesia) is associated with:**
  a. Topotecan
  b. Paclitaxel
  c. Carboplatin
  d. Liposomal doxorubicin

39. **Immunostaining positive for typical of primary ovarian cancer is:**
  a. SATB2
  b. CK20
  c. CEA
  d. PAX8

40. **Poly (ADP-ribose) polymerase (PARP) inhibitor used in ovarian cancer includes all, *except*:**
  a. Sorafenib
  b. Rucaparib
  c. Olaparib
  d. Niraparib

41. In ovarian cancer surgery; optimal cytoreduction means:

a. Residual disease < 0.5 cm
b. Residual disease < 1 cm
c. Residual disease < 1.5 cm
d. Residual disease < 2 cm

42. True about clear cell ovarian cancer includes all, *except*:

a. May arise from endometriosis
b. Napsin A positive
c. WT1 negative
d. Estrogen receptor (ER) positive

43. Endometrioid ovarian cancer is positive for all, *except*:

a. Cytokeratin 7 (CK7)
b. PAX8
c. CA125
d. CK20

44. As per World Health Organization (WHO) classification; following are considered benign ovarian tumors, *except*:

a. Brenner tumor
b. Mature teratoma
c. Signet-ring stromal tumor
d. Mesothelioma

45. As per WHO classification; following are considered borderline ovarian tumors, *except*:

a. Gonadoblastoma
b. Plasmacytoma
c. Strumal carcinoid
d. Juvenile granulosa cell tumor

46. As per WHO classification; following are considered borderline ovarian tumors, *except*:

a. Cellular fibroma
b. Mixed germ cell—sex cord—stromal tumor
c. Sertoli cell tumor
d. Mixed germ cell tumor

47. True about mucinous ovarian carcinomas includes all, *except*:

a. 71% are from metastasis from gastrointestinal tracts
b. 29% are of primary mucinous ovarian cancers
c. Mostly high grade
d. Elevated CA19-9 and carcinoembryonic antigen (CEA) levels

48. Age-adjusted mortality rate of ovarian cancer per 100,000 women is:

a. 3.4
b. 4.5
c. 5.4
d. 7.4

49. Increased relative risk of ovarian cancer is associated with all, *except*:

a. Early menarche
b. Late menopause
c. History of hysterectomy or tubal ligation
d. Nulliparity

50. True about risk reduction chemoprevention in ovarian cancer by OCP is:

a. Persists up to 5 years after discontinuation of use
b. Protection offered is around 90%
c. Level of protection is related to duration of use
d. Depends upon the age of the patient

51. All are true about risk reduction chemoprevention in ovarian cancer by OCP, *except*:

a. Applies to both nulliparity and multiparity
b. Independent of age
c. Applies to all histologic subtypes
d. Inconsistent across different races

52. Surgical procedures offering protection from ovarian cancer are:

a. Prophylactic bilateral salpingo-oophorectomy
b. Bilateral radical fimbriectomy
c. Opportunistic bilateral salpingectomy
d. Bilateral tubal ligation
e. All of the above

ANSWERS KEY

1. a	2. c	3. a	4. d	5. d	6. c	7. d
8. b	9. a	10. d	11. b	12. a	13. b	14. c
15. d	16. b	17. a	18. a	19. c	20. d	21. b
22. a	23. d	24. d	25. a	26. c	27. b	28. d
29. a	30. a	31. d	32. d	33. d	34. c	35. a
36. b	37. b	38. d	39. d	40. a	41. b	42. d
43. d	44. d	45. b	46. d	47. c	48. d	49. c
50. c	51. d	52. e				

NOTES: EPITHELIAL OVARIAN CANCER

- *Origin of epithelial ovarian cancer*: Proposed theories are:
  - Fimbriated end of fallopian tube
  - Endosalpingiosis (implantation of fallopian tube secretory cells into ovarian surface epithelium following ovulation)
  - Inclusion cysts beneath the ovarian surface
- *Dualistic model of epithelial ovarian carcinogenesis (Kurman, 2008)*:
  - *Type I*:
    - Low grade, confined to ovary, and excellent prognosis.
    - Arise from ovarian surface epithelium and mullerian inclusions by endosalpingiosis or invagination of the ovarian surface epithelium during repair following ovulation. They can also arise from implantation of cells from the endometriosis.
    - Examples are low grade serous, endometrioid, clear cell, and mucinous carcinomas (heterogenous group).
  - *Type II*:
    - Usually advanced stage and is associated with p53 mutations and poor prognosis.
    - Resembles the fallopian tube mucosa. Serous tubal intraepithelial carcinomas (STIC) is a precursor of high grade serous carcinoma (HGSC).
    - Examples are HGSC, carcinosarcomas, and undifferentiated carcinomas.
- *Types of invasive epithelial ovarian cancer*:
  - Serous (75–80%)
  - Mucinous (10%)
  - Endometrioid (10%)
  - Clear cell
  - Brenner
  - Undifferentiated
- Borderline tumors are usually confined to the ovary in premenopausal women and with good prognosis. Invasive or noninvasive peritoneal implants may also be present. The principal treatment of borderline ovarian tumors is surgical resection of the primary tumor. Conservative management in the form of fertility-sparing surgery (unilateral salpingo-oophorectomy) may also be offered. The recurrence rate after fertility-sparing surgery is around 18.5–4.6% after nonfertility sparing surgery.
- Low-grade serous cancer (LGSC) comprises approximately 5% of all epithelial cancers. They are clinically and molecularly distinct subtypes and similar to the borderline ovarian tumors. LGSCs are diagnosed at a younger age than HGSC and are usually at advance staged at presentation.
- There is no proven effective method of screening for ovarian cancer. Clinical examination, CA125, and transvaginal sonography are not effective as screening.

- Hereditary nonpolyposis colorectal cancer (HNPCC) or Lynch syndrome: Risk of ovarian cancer is 8%.
- *Prognostic variables in early-staged epithelial ovarian cancer:*
  - *Low risk:* Low grade, intact capsule, no surface excrescences, no ascites, no dense adhesions, no intraoperative rupture, negative peritoneal cytology, and diploid tumors.
  - *High-risk:* High grade, surface excrescences, tumor growth through capsule, ascites, preoperative rupture, malignant cells in ascites, dense adherence, and aneuploid tumor.
- *Preoperative assessment for optimal cytoreduction:*
  - CA125 < 500 can predict the possibility of optimal cytoreduction.
  - CT scan findings of peritoneal thickening and ascites has been associated with 32% optimal cytoreduction (the accuracy of CT scan in predicting suboptimal cytoreduction dropped to as low as 34%).
  - Fagotti score is based upon the presence of omental disease, peritoneal and diaphragmatic carcinomatosis, mesenteric involvement, bowel and stomach infiltration, and liver metastasis. It is used to select patients for either primary surgery with the aim of complete cytoreduction or for neoadjuvant chemotherapy. The positive predictive value was reported to be 100% for patients with a score >8.
- *Benefits of primary cytoreductive surgery:*
  - Physiologic benefits of tumor excision
  - Improved tumor perfusion
- *Optimal cytoreduction to <1 cm maximum residual disease depends upon:*
  - Surgery by an aggressive surgeon
  - Presence of carcinomatosis
  - American Society of Anesthesiologists (ASA) score
- Histologic type and grade of the tumor is not a prognostic factor (stage for stage). Exception to this rule include Clear Cell and Mucinous carcinomas
- *Debate in between primary cytoreductive surgery versus neoadjuvant chemotherapy (NACT):* CHORUS trial and SCORPION trial.
- *Use of liposomal doxorubicin:* CALYPSO trial.
- *Role of secondary cytoreductive surgery:* DESKTOP trial.
- *Role of bevacizumab:* Trials include OCEANS, GOG 214, and AURELIA.
- *Role of PARP inhibitors:* Trials include SOLO, NOVA, and ARIEL.
- *Role of pembrolizumab:* KEYNOTE-100 study.
- *CHORUS Trial:* Phase 3, non-inferiority, randomized, controlled trial and enrolled women with suspected stage III or IV ovarian cancer. Neoadjuvant chemotherapy and upfront debulking surgery result in similar overall survival in advanced tubo-ovarian cancer, with better survival in women with stage IV disease with neoadjuvant chemotherapy. This pooled analysis, with long-term follow-up, shows that neoadjuvant chemotherapy is a valuable treatment option for patients with stage IIIC–IV tubo-ovarian cancer, particularly in patients with a high tumor

burden at presentation or poor performance status. In women with stage III or IV ovarian cancer, survival with primary chemotherapy is non-inferior to primary surgery.

- *SCORPION Trial*: Phase III randomized clinical trial comparing primary surgery versus neoadjuvant chemotherapy in advanced epithelial ovarian cancer with high tumor. Perioperative moderate/severe morbidity were lower in neoadjuvant chemotherapy (NACT)/interval debulking surgery (IDS) arm than primary debulking surgery (PDS) arm. Quality of life scores were more favorable in NACT/IDS arm than PDS arm.
- *DESKTOP III*: First prospectively randomized surgical and superiority trial showing an overall survival benefit of debulking surgery in recurrent ovarian cancer and highlights Importance of complete resection in recurrent ovarian cancer
  - Patients with recurrent ovarian cancer and a platinum-free interval longer than 6 months, Eastern Cooperative Oncology Group performance score of 0, ascites ≤ 500 mL, and complete resection at initial surgery. The platinum-free interval exceeded 12 months in 75% of patients. Among the 206 patients randomized to surgery, 187 were ultimately operated on, and complete resection was achieved in 75%. Almost 90% of patients received platinum-containing second-line chemotherapy in both arms of the trial. Median overall survival in the intent-to-treat population was 53.7 months with and 46.0 months without surgery. Median progression free survival was 18.4 months with surgery and 14.0 months without surgery.
- *SOLO 1*: Maintenance olaparib in patients with newly diagnosed advanced ovarian cancer. The use of maintenance therapy with olaparib provided a substantial benefit with regard to progression-free survival among women with newly diagnosed advanced ovarian cancer and a BRCA1/2 mutation, with a 70% lower risk of disease progression or death with olaparib than with placebo.
- *SOLO 1*: SOLO 2 showed that maintenance therapy with the PARP inhibitor olaparib in pts with platinum-sensitive relapsed ovarian cancer and a BRCA mutation led to a statistically significant improvement in median progression-free survival of 13.6 months vs placebo.
- *SOLO 3*: Randomized phase III trial on 266 gBRCA mutated platinum sensitive relapsed ovarian cancer patients, comparing olaparib tablets (300 mg BID) versus non platinum treatment (weekly paclitaxel, weekly topotecan, gemcitabine, or pegylated liposomal doxorubicin). The overall response rate and the progression free survival favored Olaparib. At present, no mature overall data are available, while quality of life did not report any difference between the two treatment arms.

Germ Cell Ovarian Tumors and Sex Cord-Stromal Tumors

1. Lactic dehydrogenase (LDH) is increased in:

a. Dysgerminoma

b. Immature teratoma

c. Endodermal sinus tumor

d. All of the above

2. Placental alkaline phosphatase is increased in:

a. Dysgerminoma

b. Immature teratoma

c. Endodermal sinus tumor

d. All of the above

3. Alpha-fetoprotein (AFP) is increased in:

a. Embryonal carcinoma

b. Immature teratoma

c. Endodermal sinus tumor

d. All of the above

4. Percentage of germ cell ovarian tumor in first two decades of life is:

a. 40%

b. 50%

c. 60%

d. 70%

5. Human chorionic gonadotropin (hCG) is elevated in:

a. Choriocarcinoma

b. Embryonal carcinoma

c. Dysgerminoma

d. All of the above

6. Most common malignant germ cell tumor is:

a. Endodermal sinus tumor

b. Immature teratoma

c. Dysgerminoma

d. Mixed germ cell tumor

7. Percentage of dysgerminoma associated with phenotypic females with abnormal gonads is:

a. 5%

b. 10%

c. 15%

d. 20%

8. Percentage of dysgerminoma being bilateral (both gross and microscopic) is:

a. 5–10%

b. 10–15%

c. 10–20%

d. <5%

9. True about dysgerminoma includes all, *except*:

a. Periodic acid-Schiff (PAS) stain positive

b. c-kit staining

    c. Placental-like alkaline phosphatase (PLAP) positive
    d. CD30 positive

10. **Most common site of metastasis in dysgerminoma is:**
    a. Lower vertebrae
    b. Lung
    c. Liver
    d. Para-aortic lymph nodes

11. **Most commonly used chemotherapy "BEP" used in germ cell ovarian malignancy is:**
    a. Bleomycin
    b. Etoposide
    c. Cisplatin
    d. Cyclophosphamide

12. **Recurrences in dysgerminoma are associated with all, *except*:**
    a. Tumor size >15 cm diameter
    b. Age >20 years
    c. Increased mitotic factor
    d. Medullary pattern

13. **Grading of ovarian immature teratomas is based upon:**
    a. LVSI component
    b. AFP level
    c. Neuroepithelium component
    d. Glial implants

14. **Most common site of metastasis in immature teratoma is:**
    a. Lower vertebrae
    b. Peritoneum
    c. Liver
    d. Retroperitoneum lymph node

15. **Most important prognostic factor in case of immature teratoma is:**
    a. Age of the patient
    b. Grade of the lesion
    c. Nodal involvement
    d. Tumor marker level

16. **True about endodermal sinus tumor (yolk sac tumor) includes all, *except*:**
    a. Secretes AFP and alpha-1-antitrypsin
    b. Limited surgical staging in the form of unilateral salpingo-oophorectomy
    c. Chemotherapy should be given to all after the primary surgery
    d. Mostly as bilateral ovarian tumor

17. **True about yolk sac tumor includes all, *except*:**
    a. Second most common ovarian germ cell tumor
    b. Grow very slowly
    c. Abundant hemorrhage and necrosis with gelatinous material
    d. Mostly unilateral

18. **Alpha-fetoprotein level is increased in all, *except*:**
    a. Immature teratoma
    b. Embryonal carcinoma
    c. Mixed germ cell tumor
    d. Dysgerminoma

19. **Most common component of mixed germ cell tumor is:**

    a. Endodermal sinus tumor   b. Embryonal carcinoma

    c. Immature teratoma   d. Dysgerminoma

20. **Chances of recurrences after surgery in stage I ovarian germ cell tumor with adjuvant chemotherapy are:**

    a. 20–30%   b. 10–20%

    c. 10–15%   d. 5–10%

21. **Most common ovarian sex cord-stromal tumor is:**

    a. Granulosa cell tumor   b. Sertoli–Leydig cell tumor

    c. Thecoma fibroma   d. Fibroma

22. **Most common malignant ovarian sex cord-stromal tumor is:**

    a. Granulosa cell tumor   b. Sertoli–Leydig cell tumor

    c. Thecoma fibroma   d. Fibroma

23. **Juvenile granulosa cell tumor most commonly presents as:**

    a. Isosexual precocious pseudopuberty

    b. Maffucci's syndrome

    c. Ollier's disease

    d. Leprechaunism

24. **Granulosa cell tumor includes all, *except*:**

    a. Mutation involved in FOXL2402CG

    b. Endometrial cancer association in 5% cases

    c. 25% cases are associated with isosexual pseudoprecocity

    d. Endometrial hyperplasia association in 50% cases

25. **Markers of granulosa cell tumor include:**

    a. Inhibin B   b. Estrogen

    c. AMH   d. CD99

    e. All of the above

26. **Predictors of early recurrence in granulosa cell tumor include all, *except*:**

    a. Presence of residual disease   b. Presence of Call-Exner bodies

    c. DNA ploidy   d. Mitotic rate

27. **Granulosa cell tumor includes all, *except*:**

    a. Juvenile GCT is more aggressive than adult GCT

    b. Absence of Call-Exner bodies is a predictor of early recurrence

    c. Bilateral in 2% cases

    d. None of the above

28. Most important prognostic factor in adult granulosa cell tumor is:

a. Mitotic activity
b. Tumor size
c. Surgical stage
d. Tumor rupture

29. Most common lymphoma associated with ovarian cancer includes:

a. Burkitt lymphoma
b. Mantle cell lymphoma
c. T-cell lymphoma
d. Follicular lymphoma

30. Paraneoplastic hypercalcemia is associated with ovarian malignancy.

a. Carcinoid tumor
b. Lipoid cell tumor
c. Krukenberg tumor
d. Small cell carcinomas

31. Sertoli–Leydig cell tumor is associated with virilization in:

a. 80%
b. 50%
c. 30%
d. 10%

32. Incidence of Sertoli–Leydig tumors below 40 years is:

a. 10%
b. 30%
c. 50%
d. 75%

33. Adenocarcinoma of ovary and endometrium can coexist in:

a. 2%
b. 5%
c. 10%
d. None of the above

34. What percentage of ovarian tumors are metastatic from other organs?

a. 1%
b. 5%
c. 8%
d. 10%

35. What percentage of primary ovarian carcinoid tumor is associated with carcinoid syndrome?

a. 5%
b. 30%
c. 50%
d. 100%

ANSWERS KEY

1. a	2. a	3. d	4. d	5. d	6. c	7. a
8. c	9. d	10. d	11. d	12. b	13. c	14. b
15. b	16. d	17. b	18. d	19. b	20. a	21. d
22. a	23. a	24. c	25. e	26. b	27. a	28. c
29. a	30. d	31. a	32. d	33. b	34. b	35. b

NOTES: GERM CELL OVARIAN CANCER

- Nonepithelial malignancies of the ovary account for approximately 10% of all ovarian cancers.
- Germ cell tumors are derived from the primordial germ cells of the ovary. They are a model of curable cancer. About 20–25% of all benign and malignant ovarian neoplasm are of germ cell origin but they account for only about 5% of all malignant ovarian neoplasms.
- Germ cell malignant tumors grow very rapidly and are often characterized by subacute pelvic pain (hemorrhage/necrosis/distension).
- All premenarchal girls with malignant germ cell tumors should be offered karyotyping because of the chances of dysgenetic gonads.
- *Classification of germ cell tumor according to prognosis:*
  - Good (3-year progression free survival 88%)
  - Intermediate (3-year progression free survival 78%)
  - Poor-risk (3-year progression free survival 31%)
- *World Health Organization (WHO)'s histologic subtypes of germ cell tumor:*
  - *Primitive germ cell tumor:*
    - Dysgerminoma yolk sac tumor
    - Embryonal carcinoma polyembryoma
    - Nongestational choriocarcinoma
    - Mixed germ cell tumor
  - *Biphasic or triphasic teratoma:*
    - Immature teratoma
    - Mature teratoma (solid/cystic/fetiform teratoma/dermoid cyst)
  - *Monodermal teratoma:*
    - Struma ovarii (benign/malignant) carcinoid
    - Neuroectodermal tumor
    - Melanocytic sebaceous/pituitary-type tumor
- Dysgerminoma is the most common type of malignant germ cell tumor and it affects approximately 30–40% of ovarian germ cell tumors. Approximately, 65% of dysgerminoma are stage I at the diagnosis.
- Surgery of choice in case of dysgerminoma is unilateral salpingo-oophorectomy even in the presence of metastatic disease because it is very sensitive to platinum-based chemotherapy. Contralateral ovary should be removed in case of a Y-karyotype. Most common chemotherapeutic agents used are BEP (bleomycin, etoposide and cisplatin). Recurrences are uncommon and the most common sites are the peritoneal cavity and the pelvic/para-aortic lymph nodes.
- *Toxicity of BEP regimes:* Raynaud's phenomenon, neuropathy, hearing loss, tinnitus, pulmonary toxicity, acute myeloid leukemia or myelodysplastic syndrome, hypertension, and renal impairment. Hence, maximum 3–4 doses of BEP are only given.

- Transient ovarian failure may occur with BEP, but in most of the cases there is resumption of ovarian functions after the completion of the chemotherapy.
- Immature teratoma is the second most common malignant germ cell tumor of the ovary.
- Prognosis of immature teratoma depends upon the amount of immature neuroepithelial cells present in the tumor. The most important prognostic factors in case of immature teratoma are the stage and grade of the tumor.
- Squamous cell carcinoma is the most common type of malignant transformation seen in case of mature teratoma.
- Endodermal sinus tumors are the third most common malignant germ cell tumor of the ovary. It secretes AFP.
- Sex-cord stromal tumor account for 5–8% of all the ovarian malignancies.
- *WHO classification of the sex cord-stromal tumors of the ovary*:
  - Sex-cord-stromal cell tumor
  - Granulosa cell tumor (adult and juvenile)
  - Thecoma-fibroma group (thecoma/fibroma/fibrosarcoma/sclerosing/signet-ring/unclassified)
  - Sertoli–Leydig cell tumor
  - Well/intermediate/poorly-differentiated types
  - Steroid cell tumor (stromal luteoma)
- Granulosa cell tumor is a low-grade malignant tumor and are usually confined to one ovary at the time of diagnosis. 75% of these tumors are associated with sexual pseudo precocity. Juvenile granulosa cell tumor is usually less aggressive in nature.
- *Prognostic markers of adult granulosa cell tumor*: Cellular atypia, mitotic rate, absence of Call-Exner bodies, DNA ploidy and presence of residual disease.
- Late recurrences can be there in case of granulosa cell tumor. They are 30% estrogen receptor positive and 100% progesterone receptor positive tumors. Treatment response to luteinizing hormone-releasing hormone (LHRH) agonists and aromatase inhibitors is about 50% in both the treatment groups.
- Thecoma-fibroma group are usually benign and rarely may be malignant like fibrosarcomas.
- Sertoli–Leydig tumors are usually found below 40 years age and are low-grade malignancies. They are bilateral in <1% cases. Recurrences are uncommon.
- Malignant mixed mesodermal tumors (MMMTs) have got monoclonal origin of both epithelial and sarcomatous components. Cytoreductive surgery followed by platinum-based adjuvant chemotherapy.

- Small cell carcinomas of hypercalcemic type are associated with SMARCA4 mutation. They have been recently designated as Rhabdoid tumor of the ovary.
- Krukenberg tumor is characterized by mucin-filled signet-ring cells in the ovarian stroma. They account for 30–40% of the metastatic cancers to the ovary are Krukenberg tumors and most common primary tumor is from the stomach. Most common non-Krukenberg metastatic ovarian tumor is from colon.

Vulval Cancer

1. Percentage of vulval cancers due to human papillomavirus (HPV) is:

a. 70%

b. 60%

c. 50%

d. 40%

2. Most common HPV causing vulval cancer is:

a. HPV 16

b. HPV 18

c. HPV 31

d. HPV 33

3. Truth about recent changes in vulval cancer is all, *except*:

a. Use of separate groin incision for lymphadenectomy

b. Groin dissection omitted in T1 tumor with <1 mm stromal invasion

c. Early diagnosis

d. Use of sentinel lymph node biopsy

4. Association of lichen sclerosus and vulval cancer is:

a. 8%

b. 18%

c. 28%

d. 38%

5. Risk of malignancy in differentiated vulval intraepithelial neoplasia (VIN) is:

a. 85%

b. 75%

c. 35%

d. 25%

6. Risk of malignancy in usual type VIN is:

a. 85%

b. 75%

c. 35%

d. 25%

7. Paget's disease of vulva includes all, *except*:

a. Most common extra mammary site

b. Should be screened for associated malignancy

c. Histologic extent correlates well with the macroscopic lesion

d. Late recurrences

8. Immunohistochemistry in melanoma is positive for:

a. S-100

b. HMB-45

c. Melan-A

d. All of the above

9. **Buschke–Lowenstein giant condyloma is a variant of:**

a. Basal cell carcinoma
b. Verrucous carcinoma
c. Squamous cell carcinoma
d. Merkel cell tumor

10. **True about vulval verrucous carcinoma includes all, *except*:**

a. Well-differentiated type
b. Hyperkeratotic
c. Good prognosis
d. HPV related

11. **Vulval basal cell carcinoma includes all, *except*:**

a. Elderly women
b. Small diameter lesion
c. Usually in labia majora
d. HPV related

12. **Secondary Paget's disease of vulva is positive for:**

a. Uroplakin 3
b. S-100
c. HMB-35
d. Melan-A

13. **Overall incidence of groin lymph node metastasis in vulval cancer is:**

a. 40%
b. 30%
c. 20%
d. 10%

14. **Overall incidence of pelvic lymph node metastasis in vulval cancer is:**

a. 9%
b. 18%
c. 28%
d. 30%

15. **Percentage of positive pelvic lymph nodes in presence of positive groin lymph nodes is:**

a. 10%
b. 20%
c. 30%
d. 50%

16. **A vulval cancer lesion of size 3 cm involving lower one-third vagina and one positive inguinofemoral lymph node:**

a. Stage III A
b. Stage III B
c. Stage III C
d. Stage II

17. **During the management of the primary vulval lesions, the incidence of local invasive recurrence is low if the surgical margin is at least:**

a. 1 cm
b. 1.5 cm
c. 2 cm
d. 2.5 cm

18. **During the management of the primary vulval lesions, the incidence of local invasive recurrence is low if the histological margin is at least:**

a. 8 mm
b. 10 mm
c. 15 mm
d. 20 mm

19. Indication of groin lymph node dissection includes all, *except*:

a. Lesion size of 2 cm and stromal invasion > 1 mm
b. Lesion size > 2 cm diameter
c. Lesion size ≤ 2 cm and stromal invasion < 1 mm
d. All of the above

20. Indication of unilateral inguino-femoral lymphadenectomy include:

a. Involvement of anterior labia minora
b. Ipsilateral negative lymph node
c. Lesion is within 2 cm from the midline
d. All of the above

21. The average difference between tumor thickness and depth of invasion is (Wilkinson method):

a. 0.3 mm
b. 0.4 mm
c. 0.6 mm
d. 0.8 mm

22. True about groin lymph node anatomy includes:

a. No lymph node adjacent to anterior superior iliac spine
b. Femoral lymph nodes are always medial to the femoral vein
c. Cloquet lymph node is inconsistent
d. All of the above

23. Following groin lymph node dissection, chronic lower limb lymphedema occurs in:

a. 30%
b. 40%
c. 50%
d. 60%

24. Following groin lymph node dissection, early postoperative lymphocyst formation occurs in:

a. 30%
b. 40%
c. 50%
d. 60%

25. Percentage of false-negative sentinel lymph node in vulval cancer:

a. 2% to 3%
b. 5% to 10%
c. 10% to 15%
d. 15% to 20%

26. Indication of bilateral groin and pelvic radiation in vulval cancer includes:

a. ≥3 micrometastases
b. One macrometastasis
c. Extracapsular involvement of lymph node
d. All of the above

27. Significant prognostic variables in vulval cancer includes all, *except*:
 a. ECOG performance status
 b. Number of positive groin lymph nodes
 c. Extracapsular lymph node involvement
 d. Age of the patient

28. With the appropriate curative intent of management, vulval cancer has got an overall 5-year survival rate of:
 a. 60%
 b. 65%
 c. 70%
 d. 75%

29. True about vulval melanoma include all, *except*:
 a. Prognosis depends upon the diameter of the lesion
 b. Prognosis depends upon the depth of involvement
 c. Most common location is labia minora or clitoris
 d. Prognosis depends upon the lymph node status

30. Honan's criteria are used for:
 a. Urethral cancer
 b. Bartholin gland carcinoma
 c. Vulval schwannoma
 d. Vulval melanoma

31. Rodent ulcer in vulva is:
 a. Verrucous carcinoma
 b. Vulvar sarcoma
 c. Vulvar adenocarcinoma
 d. 31 basal cell carcinoma

32. As per National Comprehensive Cancer Network (NCCN) guidelines workup for a case of vulvar cancer include:
 a. HIV testing
 b. HPV testing
 c. Smoking cessation
 d. All of the above

33. In stage IB II vulval cancer: percentage of inguinofemoral lymph node metastasis is:
 a. >5%
 b. >8%
 c. >15%
 d. >20%

34. Risk of contralateral metastasis in a negative unilateral inguino-femoral lymph node dissection:
 a. <3%
 b. <5%
 c. <8%
 d. <10%

35. Risk of lymphatic metastasis in stage IA vulval cancer with clinically negative nodes is:
 a. <0.5%
 b. <1%
 c. <3%
 d. <5%

36. **True about radical local excision and radical vulvectomy includes all, *except*:**

a. Depth of resection is more in radical vulvectomy
b. No difference in terms of recurrence in between the two surgeries
c. Depth of resection is not defined in radical local excision
d. No prospective comparison trial between the two techniques of surgeries till date

37. **Most important prognostic factor in vulval cancer is:**

a. Status of the inguinofemoral lymph nodes
b. Tumor diameter
c. Tumor thickness
d. Grade of the tumor

38. **Adverse prognostic factor in vulval cancer is:**

a. DNA ploidy
b. Tumor volume
c. Proliferative index
d. Margin status

39. **Most adverse prognostic factor in vulval cancer is:**

a. p53 overexpression
b. Association with VIN
c. Ulceration and keratin content
d. Depth of invasion

40. **Adverse prognostic factor in vulval cancer includes all, *except*:**

a. Tumor diameter
b. Tumor thickness
c. LVSI
d. Tumor growth pattern

41. **Adverse prognostic factor in vulval cancer includes all, *except*:**

a. Tumor diameter
b. Tumor margin
c. Tumor thickness
d. Tumor grade

42. **Lymph node prognostic factor of vulval cancer includes:**

a. Bilateral involvement
b. Extracapsular involvement
c. Location of metastasis within the node
d. Number of lymph nodes involved
e. All of the above

43. **Most common HPV causing vulvar cancer is:**

a. HPV 16
b. HPV 18
c. HPV 33
d. HPV 11

44. **Vulval cancer accounts for what percentage of total gynecological malignancies in the world?**

a. 4%
b. 10%
c. 15%
d. 2%

ANSWERS KEY

1. d	2. a	3. c	4. c	5. a	6. d	7. c
8. d	9. b	10. d	11. d	12. a	13. b	14. a
15. b	16. a	17. a	18. a	19. c	20. c	21. a
22. d	23. d	24. b	25. b	26. a	27. d	28. c
29. a	30. b	31. d	32. d	33. b	34. a	35. b
36. a	37. a	38. a	39. d	40. d	41. d	42. d
43. e	44. a					

NOTES: VULVAL CANCER

- There is increase in the incidence of VIN and vulvar cancer in the recent times. The increased incidence in younger women has been attributed to changing sexual behavior, HPV infection, and cigarette smoking.
- Primary Paget's disease is positive for diastase periodic acid Schiff (PASD) and mucicarmine. Only secondary Paget's disease of vulva of urothelial origin is positive for Uroplakin 3.
- Approximately 40% of vulvar cancers are HPV positive and 85% of HPV positive invasive vulvar cancers are attributable to HPV-16.
- *Spread of the vulvar cancer can be*: Direct, lymphatic, and hematogenous. Lymphatic spread to the inguinal lymph nodes may occur early. Metastasis to the femoral nodes without the involvement of the inguinal nodes may also occur.
- Treatment of vulvar cancer is individualized and takes into consideration the primary lesion and the groin lymph node management separately. Primary lesion may be unifocal or multifocal. The unaffected part of the vulva and the affected part of the vulva including the involvement/ proximity of the clitoris, urethra, vagina, and anus are important surgical considerations.
- Radicality of the surgery involves a wide and deep surgical approach. Surgical approach should be advocated whenever, there is a chance of getting a negative surgical margin. Surgical approaches for the primary lesion include wide local excision, radical vulvectomy, and radical hemivulvectomy.
- Complications of radical vulvectomy include urinary stress incontinence, genital prolapse, introital stenosis, and pubic osteomyelitis.

- *Closure of large defects*:
  - Gracilis myocutaneous grafts
  - Transverse rectus abdominis muscle myocutaneous (TRAM) graft
  - Advancement flaps (V-Y gluteal fold or medial thigh flap)
  - Transpositional flaps (lotus petal, gluteal/anterolateral thigh flap, and angel wing perforator-based island flap)
- Vulvar cancer may be considered to be advanced if it is unresectable or marginally resectable because of the involvement of the vagina, anus, urethra, or other adjacent structures, or if there are bulky lymph node metastasis.
- Patients without significant risk of lymph node metastasis are those with a tumor size ≤2 cm in diameter and that invades the stroma to a depth <1 mm. Patients who develop recurrences in an undissected groin have a very high mortality rate.
- Surgical approach to a lymph node dissection is a thorough inguino-femoral lymphadenectomy. Bilateral groin dissection may be avoided when the primary lesion is unilateral (defined as 2 cm or more from the midline) and the ipsilateral nodes are negative. Bilateral groin dissections should be done when the lesions involve the anterior labia minora. Complications of lymphadenectomy include lymphocyst formation, cellulitis, and chronic lower limb lymphedema.
- False negative rate of the sentinel node procedure as per various studies is agreed to be around 5%.
- *GROINS-V*: Groningen International Study is based on sentinel nodes in vulvar cancer.
- *GROINS-V I* stated that the recurrence rates were similar for those having sentinel lymph node biopsy or lymphadenectomy. If the sentinel lymph node is positive then additional groin treatment is mandatory. There was no cut-off in the size of the metastatic focus in the sentinel lymph node.
- *GROINS-V II* result states that inguinofemoral radiotherapy is a safe alternative to inguinofemoral lymphadenectomy with sentinel lymph node micro-metastasis. But for patients with sentinel lymph node macro-metastasis; radiotherapy (50 Gy) resulted into more isolated groin recurrences than a inguino-femoral lymphadenectomy.
- *GROINSS-V III* will investigate whether the efficacy of treatment can be increased by adding concurrent chemotherapy to inguinofemoral radiotherapy and also increasing the total dose from 50 Gy to 56 Gy by applying a simultaneous integrated boost dose (radiotherapy dose escalation in combination with chemotherapy will be investigated in GROINSS- V III).
- *When there are clinically or radiologically suspicious lymph nodes*: Approaches include full inguinofemoral lymphadenectomy or removing only the enlarged groin nodes followed by adjuvant radiation.
- Fixed and unresectable groin nodes are treated primarily by radiation ± chemotherapy.

- Definitive preoperative radiation ± concurrent chemotherapy should be regarded as the treatment of choice for patients with advanced vulvar cancer who would otherwise require pelvic exenteration.
- Pelvic exenteration includes infralevator exenteration (anterior/posterior/total) and it is combined with radical vulvectomy and bilateral groin dissection.
- *Role of radiation therapy in vulvar cancer:*
    - Avoidance of exenteration
    - Nodes positive after surgery
    - Positive or close surgical resection margin
    - Potential preoperative roles (small clitoral/periclitoral lesions, alternative to groin dissection in No status, or in case of grossly enlarged lymph nodes)
- *Types of local recurrences in case of vulval cancer:*
    - Primary tumor site including recurrence within 2 cm from the vulvectomy scar (poor prognosis)
    - Remote vulvar recurrence (>2 cm from the primary tumor site). It is associated with better prognosis
    - Skin bridge recurrences
- Overall 5-year survival rate in operable case of vulval cancer is 70%. Lymph node status is the most important factor.
- The number of positive lymph nodes is the single most important prognostic variable. Lymph node ratio (ratio of number of positive nodes to the number of nodes removed) has shown more accurate estimation of recurrence. Extracapsular nodal involvement and extranodal involvement are also associated with poor prognosis.
- Other prognostic factors include: Eastern Cooperative Oncology Group (ECOG) performance, overexpression of cyclooxygenase 2 (COX2), DNA ploidy and presence of HPV/p16.
- Age is not a significant prognostic variable in case of vulval cancer.
- *Vulval verrucous carcinoma:* It is a slow growing locally destructive lesion. IHC shows peculiar distribution pattern of cytokeratin AE1 and AE3. Radical excision is the treatment of choice and radiation is contraindicated due to induction of anaplastic transformation.
- Vulval melanoma is biologically very unpredictable type of cancer and the prognosis is poor. International Federation of Gynecology and Obstetrics (FIGO) staging for vulval cancer is not applicable for vulval melanoma as the lesions are smaller in dimension and that the prognosis is related to the depth of penetration rather than to the diameter of the lesion.
- Treatment of vulval melanoma: Radical local excision with 1 cm margin and inguinofemoral lymphadenectomy when the stromal invasion is >1 mm. Interferon α-2b is used as an adjuvant therapy.
- Primary carcinoma of Bartholin gland accounts for about 5% of vulval cancer. It is treated by radical resection of primary lesion and ipsilateral inguinofemoral lymphadenectomy.

- *Honan's criteria for Bartholin gland carcinoma*:
  - Tumor is in correct anatomical position
  - Tumor located deep in the labium majus
  - Intact overlying skin
  - Presence of recognizable normal gland
- *Adenosquamous carcinoma of the vulva*: Propensity for perineural invasion, lymph node metastasis, and local recurrence.
- *Basal cell carcinoma of vulva*:
  - Second most common vulval cancer
  - Slow-growing locally invasive
  - Nodal metastasis is rare
  - Basal cell carcinoma should be suspected whenever inflammatory vulval lesions are not responding to usual treatment
  - Treatment is radical local excision
- Dermatofibrosarcoma protuberans is a low-grade cutaneous malignancy. Mohs micrographic surgery is used in its management.
- Vulval germ cell tumors are usually of endodermal sinus tumors.

Miscellaneous

1. **Embryo cryopreservation includes all, *except*:**
   a. Requires ovarian stimulation
   b. Delay chemotherapy
   c. Risk of reseeding cancer
   d. Cannot be used in prepuberty

2. **Oocyte cryopreservation includes all, *except*:**
   a. Requires ovarian stimulation
   b. Delay chemotherapy
   c. Risk of reseeding cancer
   d. Cannot be used in prepuberty

3. **Ovarian tissue cryopreservation includes all, *except*:**
   a. Requires ovarian stimulation
   b. Delay chemotherapy
   c. Risk of reseeding cancer
   d. Cannot be used in prepuberty

4. **Which of the following is not advised to be used as fertility preservation technique?**
   a. Embryo cryopreservation
   b. Oocyte cryopreservation
   c. Ovarian tissue cryopreservation
   d. GnRH agonist administration

5. **Levels found to be elevated in normal pregnancy include:**
   a. Inhibin B
   b. AMH
   c. LDH
   d. CA15.3

6. **Pregnant patients may undergo laparoscopic surgery for pelvic conditions safely up to:**
   a. 16 weeks
   b. 28 weeks
   c. 22 weeks
   d. 20 weeks

7. **Stochastic risk of radiotherapy during pregnancy includes:**
   a. Microcephaly
   b. Mental retardation
   c. Fetal demise
   d. Leukemia

8. **Deterministic effects of radiotherapy during pregnancy include all, *except*:**
   a. Childhood cancer
   b. Fetal growth restrictions
   c. Fetal malformations
   d. None of the above

9. True about chemotherapy in pregnancy includes all, *except*:

a. Dose is not based on actual weight and height during pregnancy
b. Drug absorption altered due to gastric secretion and motility
c. Therapeutic concentrations of active drug may be affected by hemodynamic changes of pregnancy
d. Pharmacokinetic changes due to increased plasma volume and renal clearance

10. Which of the following has got the highest fetal plasma concentrations due to transplacental pharmacokinetics?

a. Doxorubicin
b. Paclitaxel
c. Cyclophosphamide
d. Carboplatin

11. Which of the following has got the lowest fetal plasma concentrations due to transplacental pharmacokinetics?

a. Doxorubicin
b. Paclitaxel
c. Cyclophosphamide
d. Carboplatin

12. Complications of chemotherapy during second or third trimester of pregnancy include all, *except*:

a. Low birth weight
b. Preterm births
c. Congenital malformations
d. Fetal growth restrictions

13. Tumor markers not elevated in maternal serum during normal pregnancy are all, *except*:

a. Inhibin B
b. CA15-3
c. AMH
d. LDH

14. Tumor markers elevated in maternal serum during normal pregnancy are all, *except*:

a. CA125
b. CA15-3
c. Squamous cell carcinoma antigen
d. Inhibin B

15. Laparoscopic surgery in pregnancy can be safely done up to:

a. 16 weeks
b. 20 weeks
c. 24 weeks
d. 28 weeks

16. True about cancer in pregnancy is all, *except*:

a. Chemotherapy after first trimester is safe
b. Chemotherapy followed by term delivery
c. Preterm delivery without chemotherapy
d. Episiotomy is a potential site of recurrence

17. **True about cervical intraepithelial neoplasia (CIN) in pregnancy is all, *except*:**

a. Observation is the main treatment strategy.
b. Pregnancy leads to disease progression.
c. High chances of false positivity in pap smears.
d. Colposcopy should be done at 6-weeks postpartum.

18. **Not recommended for CIN in pregnancy is:**

a. Ablation or excision
b. Prenatal colposcopy for surveillance
c. Colposcopy at 6-weeks postpartum
d. Cytology for surveillance

19. **Highest complication in management for cervical cancer in pregnancy is associated with:**

a. Conization in stage IA
b. Trachelectomy in nodes negative
c. Neoadjuvant chemotherapy and radical hysterectomy postpartum
d. Radical trachelectomy

20. **Fetal loss within 16 days of radical trachelectomy procedure is:**

a. 10%
b. 20%
c. 33%
d. 43%

21. **Chemotherapeutic agents considered unsafe in pregnancy are:**

a. Trastuzumab
b. Paclitaxel
c. 5-FU
d. Doxorubicin

22. **Chemotherapeutic agent considered unsafe in pregnancy is:**

a. Methotrexate
b. Cyclophosphamide
c. Epirubicin
d. Docetaxel

23. **Most common hematologic malignancy in pregnancy is:**

a. Hodgkin lymphoma
b. Non-Hodgkin lymphoma
c. AML
d. ALL

24. **Major sign of protein depletion includes all, *except*:**

a. Serum albumin < 3.5 mg/dL
b. Absolute lymphocyte count < $1{,}500/mm^3$
c. Serum transferrin < 150 mg/dL
d. Increased reactivity to skin test antigens

25. **Prognostic Nutritional Index (PNI) in malnutrition is:**

a. >20
b. >30
c. >40
d. >50

26. Sensitivity of patient-generated subjective global assessment for malnutrition is:

a. >60%
b. >70%
c. >80%
d. >90%

27. Refeeding syndrome associated with total parenteral nutrition (TPN) is:

a. Hypoglycemia
b. Electrolyte imbalance
c. Azotemia
d. Metabolic acidosis

28. Most common metabolic complications associated with parenteral nutrition are:

a. Hyperglycemia
b. Hypoglycemia
c. Metabolic acidosis
d. Overfeeding

29. Which of the following is true regarding intravenous leiomyomatosis?

a. Associated with 50% cases of leiomyoma
b. Benign in nature
c. Worm-like extensions involve the ovaries only.
d. Most common is brain metastasis.

30. Which is the least common type of degenerations in case of fibroid uterus?

a. Necrosis
b. Red degeneration
c. Hyaline degeneration
d. Sarcomatous degeneration

31. Most common malignancy to involve vagina secondarily from cancer of:

a. Urinary bladder
b. Rectum
c. Endometrium
d. Cervix

32. Most common vaginal cancer is:

a. Squamous cell carcinoma
b. Melanoma
c. Adenocarcinoma
d. Sarcoma

33. What percentage of patients with primary vaginal carcinoma have a history of in situ or invasive cervical cancer treated 5-years back?

a. 40%
b. 30%
c. 20%
d. 10%

34. Overall, 5-years survival rate for vaginal cancer is:

a. 42%
b. 52%
c. 62%
d. 32%

35. **Which is false about verrucous carcinoma of vagina?**
   a. Locally aggressive warty lesions
   b. Minimal tendency to metastasize
   c. Surgical excision is the treatment of choice
   d. Radiation treatment improves the outcome

36. **True about primary clear cell adenocarcinoma of vagina includes all, *except*:**
   a. In utero exposure of DES
   b. Comprises 14% of primary vaginal carcinoma
   c. OCP related
   d. Not associated with history of pregnancy

37. **Most common vaginal malignant tumor in children is:**
   a. Embryonal rhabdomyosarcoma b. Clear cell adenocarcinoma
   c. Squamous cell carcinoma   d. Adenocarcinomas

38. **What protocol is used for communicating the bad news to a patient and her relative:**
   a. DELTA   b. SPIKES
   c. CARE   d. DONE

39. **Clinical criteria for depression can be seen in how many percentages of patients newly diagnosed with ovarian cancer:**
   a. 10%   b. 20%
   c. 30%   d. 40%

40. **Overall sexual dysfunction found in patients after being treated for cancer:**
   a. 20%   b. 30%
   c. 50%   d. 90%

ANSWERS KEY

1. c	2. d	3. a	4. d	5. d	6. b	7. d
8. a	9. a	10. d	11. b	12. c	13. b	14. d
15. d	16. c	17. b	18. a	19. d	20. c	21. a
22. a	23. a	24. d	25. c	26. d	27. b	28. d
29. c	30. d	31. d	32. a	33. b	34. b	35. d
36. c	37. a	38. b	39. c	40. b		

Important Facts, Figures, and Staging in Gynecological Cancers

1. Prognostic Scoring System (Bagshawe) and FIGO (International Federation of Gynecology and Obstetrics) Staging of Gestational Trophoblastic Neoplasia (GTN) (2009):

Risk factors	*0*	*1*	*2*	*4*
Age (years)	<40	≥40	–	–
Antecedent pregnancy	Mole	Abortion	Term	–
Intervals from index pregnancy	<4	4–<7	7–<13	≥13
Pretreatment hCG (IU/mL)	$<10^3$	$10^3–<10^4$	$10^4–<10^5$	$>10^5$
Largest tumor size	3–<5 cm	≥5 cm	–	–
Site of metastasis	Lung	Kidney/spleen	GIT/liver	Brain
Number of metastasis	–	1–4	5–8	>8
Previous-failed chemotherapy	–	–	Single drug	Two or more drugs

- Prognostic scoring system: Low-risk when <7; prognostic scoring system: high-risk when ≥7
- This scoring system is not valid for intermediate trophoblastic tumors (ITT) [placental site trophoblastic tumor (PSTT) and epithelioid trophoblastic tumor (ETT)]

Staging	*Location and extent of GTN*
I	Disease confined to uterus (usually low-risk)
II	• Disease confined to adnexa, broad ligament, and vagina (genital structures) • (Prognostic scoring system: Low-risk when <7) • (Prognostic scoring system: High-risk when ≥7)
III	• Disease extends to lung ± genital tract involvement • (Prognostic scoring system: Low-risk when <7) • (Prognostic scoring system: High-risk when ≥7)
IV	All other metastatic sites (brain, GIT, liver, and kidney)

2. 2018 FIGO staging of cancer cervix:

Stage I	***Carcinoma is strictly confined to the cervix and extension to the corpus should be disregarded***
I A	I A1: Depth of stromal invasion ≤3 mm
	I A2: Depth of stromal invasion >3 mm and ≤5 mm
I B	I B1: Invasive carcinoma >5 mm depth of stromal invasion and ≤2 cm in greatest dimension
	I B2: Invasive carcinoma >2 cm and ≤4 cm in greatest dimension
	I B3: Invasive carcinoma >4 cm in greatest dimension
Stage II	***Carcinoma extended beyond the uterus but not to the lower third of the vagina/pelvic side-wall***
II A	II A1: Invasive carcinoma ≤4 cm in greatest dimension
	II A2: Invasive carcinoma >4 cm in greatest dimension
II B	With parametrial invasion but not up to the pelvic side-wall
Stage III	***Carcinoma cervix involves the lower third of the vagina/pelvic side-wall and/ or causes hydronephrosis or nonfunctioning kidney and/or involves pelvic and/or para-aortic lymph nodes***
III	III A: Carcinoma involves the lower third of the vagina with no extension to the pelvic side-wall
	III B: Carcinoma involves the pelvic side-wall or caused hydronephrosis or non functioning kidney (unless due to other known cause)
	III C1: Pelvic lymph node metastasis III C2: Para-aortic lymph node metastasis • Including micro-metastasis • Irrespective of the tumor size or extent of the disease • Notations for designation of assessment by radiology as "r" and by pathology as "p", respectively.
Stage IV	***Carcinoma extended beyond true pelvis or has involved the mucosa of bladder or rectum as proven by biopsy (bullous edema is not used to assign stage)***
IV	IV A: Spread of the disease to adjacent organs
	IV B: Spread to distant organs

Note:
- LVSI do not change the staging
- Isolated tumor cells do not change the staging
- Lateral extent of the disease in stage I A (up to 7 mm) is no longer valid in the new staging
- Type of imaging or pathology modalities used is no longer valid
- When in doubt the lower staging should be assigned.
- Ideal clinical assessment should be done under anesthesia (EUA)

3. **Type I versus type II endometrial cancer (adenocarcinoma): originally by Bookman (1983):**

Endometrial cancer	Type I	Type II
Clinical and pathological characteristics	• Young age • Early stage with favorable prognosis • Obesity, unopposed estrogen endometrioid variety • Well-differentiated variety	• Old age-advanced stage • Non-endometrioid type aggressive variety • Poorly-differentiated variety • Advanced stage on presentation
Molecular characteristics	Diploid and MSI in 35%	Aneuploid and MSI is rare
Mutations in tumor suppressor gene	*ARID1A, PTEN, MLH1, CTCF, and POLE*	*TP53, HER2/neu, FBXW7, and PPP2R1A*
Oncogene mutations/ amplifications	*PIK3CA, PIK3R1, KRAS, and CTNNB1*	*MYC and PIK3CA*

4. **2009 FIGO surgical staging for endometrial cancer:**
(**Carcinosarcomas are also staged like that of endometrial cancer)

Stage I	Tumor confined to the corpus uteri
I A	No or <50% myometrial invasion
I B	≥50% myometrial invasion
Stage II	Tumor invades cervical stroma, but does not extend beyond the uterus
Stage III	Local ± regional spread of tumor
III A	Serosal involvement and/or adnexal involvement
III B	Vaginal and/or parametrial involvement
III C	III C1: Metastasis to pelvic lymph nodes III C2: Metastasis to para-aortic lymph nodes and/or pelvic lymph nodes
Stage IV	IV A: Tumor invades bladder and/or bowel mucosa IV B: Distant metastasis including intra-abdominal metastasis and/or inguinal lymph nodes

Note:
- Each staging can further be divided into Grade 1, Grade 2 and Grade 3
- Only endocervical glandular involvement should be considered as Stage I and no longer as Stage II
- Positive cytology is reported separately

5. **2009 FIGO staging for leiomyosarcomas:**

Stage I	Tumor limited to uterus I A: <5 cm I B: >5 cm
Stage II	Tumor extends to pelvis II A: Adnexal involvement II B: Tumor extends to extrauterine pelvic tissue
Stage III	Tumor invades abdominal tissues III A: One site III B: More than one site III C: Metastasis to pelvic ± para-aortic lymph nodes
Stage IV	IV A: Tumor invades bowel and/or rectum IV B: Distant metastasis

6. 2009 FIGO staging for endometrial stromal sarcomas and adenosarcomas:

Stage I	*Limited to uterus*
I A	Tumor limited to endometrium/endocervix with no myometrial invasion
I B	≤50% myometrial invasion
I C	>50% myometrial invasion
Stage II	*Tumor extends to the pelvis*
II A	Adnexal involvement
II B	Tumor extends to extrauterine pelvic tissue
Stage III	*Tumor invades abdominal tissues*
III A	One site
III B	More than one site
III C	Metastasis to pelvic and/or para-aortic lymph nodes
Stage IV	*Regional and distant metastasis*
IV A	Tumor invades bladder and/or rectum
IV B	Distant metastasis

7. International Federation of Gynecology and Obstetrics staging of ovarian, fallopian tube, and primary peritoneal cancer (2019):

Stage I: Tumor confined to the ovaries (one or both) or fallopian tube(s)	
I A	• Tumor limited to one ovary (capsule intact) or fallopian tube, no tumor on ovarian or fallopian tube surface • No malignant cells in ascites or peritoneal washings
I B	• Tumor limited to both ovaries (capsule intact) or fallopian tube, no tumor on ovarian or fallopian tube surface • No malignant cells in ascites or peritoneal washings
I C	*Tumor limited to one or both ovaries or fallopian tubes and with any of the following:* • I C1: Surgical spill • I C2: Capsule ruptured before surgery or tumor on ovarian or fallopian tube surface • I C3: Malignant cells in ascites or peritoneal washings
Stage II: Tumor involves one or both ovaries or fallopian tubes with pelvic extension below pelvic brim or primary peritoneal cancer	
II A	Extension and/or implants on the uterus and/or fallopian tube(s) and/or ovaries
II B	Extension to and/or implants on other pelvic tissues
Stage III: Tumor involves one or both ovaries or fallopian tubes or primary peritoneal cancer with microscopically confirmed peritoneal metastasis outside the pelvis and/or metastasis to the retroperitoneal (pelvic and/or para-aortic) lymph nodes	
III A1	*Histologically confirmed positive retroperitoneal lymph nodes:* III A1 (i) metastasis ≤ 10 mm in greatest dimension III A1 (ii) metastasis > 10 mm in greatest dimension

Contd...

Contd…

III A2	Microscopic extra-pelvic (above pelvic brim) peritoneal involvement with or without positive retroperitoneal lymph nodes
III B	Macroscopic peritoneal metastasis beyond pelvis ≤2 cm or less in greatest dimension with or without metastasis to the retroperitoneal lymph nodes
III C	Macroscopic peritoneal metastasis beyond the pelvis >2 cm in greatest dimension with or without metastasis to the retroperitoneal lymph nodes (includes extension of tumor to capsule of liver and spleen without parenchymal involvement of either organ
Stage IV: Distant metastasis including pleural effusion with positive cytology/liver or splenic parenchymal metastasis/metastasis to extra-abdominal organs (inguinal nodes or nodes outside the abdominal cavity)/transmural involvement of intestine	
IV A	Pleural effusion with positive cytology
IV B	Liver or splenic parenchymal metastasis/metastasis to extra-abdominal organs (inguinal nodes or nodes outside the abdominal cavity)/transmural involvement of intestine

8. International Federation of Gynecology and Obstetrics staging of vulval cancer (2009):

Stage I: Tumor confined to the vulva and/or perineum and with negative nodes	
Depth of invasion: Measurement of the tumor from the epithelial-stromal junction of the adjacent most superficial dermal papilla to the deepest point of invasion	
I A	Lesions ≤ 2 cm and stromal invasion ≤ 1 mm
I B	Lesions > 2 cm or stromal invasion > 1 mm
Stage II: Tumor of any size with extension to adjacent perineal structures with negative nodes (one-third lower urethra, one-third lower vagina, and anus)	
Stage III: Tumor of any size with extension to adjacent perineal structures with positive nodes (one-third lower urethra, one-third lower vagina, and anus) with positive inguinal femoral lymph nodes	
III A	1–2 lymph node metastasis (<5 mm) or 1 lymph node metastasis (≥5 mm)
III B	≥3 lymph node metastasis (<5 mm) or ≥2 lymph node metastasis (≥5 mm)
III C	Positive lymph nodes with extracapsular spread
Stage IV: Tumor invades other regional (two-thirds upper urethra and two-thirds upper vagina) or distant metastasis	
IV A	Tumor involves upper urethra/vaginal mucosa or bladder mucosa/rectal mucosa or fixed to the pelvic bone or with fixed/ulcerated inguinofemoral lymph nodes
IV B	Any distant metastasis including pelvic lymph nodes

New FIGO (2021) Staging for Vulval Cancer

Stage I: Tumor confined to the vulva and/or perineum and with negative nodes Depth of invasion is measured from the basement membrane of the deepest, adjacent, dysplastic, tumor-free rete ridge (or nearest dysplastic rete peg) to the deepest point of invasion.	
I A	Lesions ≤ 2 cm and stromal invasion ≤ 1 mm
I B	Lesions > 2 cm or stromal invasion > 1 mm
Stage II: Tumor of any size with extension to lower 1/3rd urethra, lower 1/3rd vagina, lower 1/3rd anus with negative nodes	
Stage III: Tumor of any size with extension to the upper part of adjacent perineal structures, or with any number of non-fixed, nonulcerated lymph node	
III A	Tumor of any size with disease extension to upper 2/3rd of urethra, upper 2/3rd of vagina, bladder mucosa, rectal mucosa, or regional lymph node metastasis ≤ 5 mm
III B	Regional (inguinal and femoral) lymph node metastasis > 5 mm
III C	Regional (inguinal and femoral) lymph node metastasis with extra-capsular spread
Stage IV: Tumor of any size fixed to bone, or fixed, ulcerated lymph node metastasis, or distant metastasis	
IV A	Disease fixed to pelvic bone, or fixed or ulcerated regional (inguinal and femoral) lymph node metastasis
IV B	Distant metastasis

9. International Federation of Gynecology and Obstetrics staging of vaginal cancer (2009):

Stage I: Carcinoma is limited to the vaginal wall	
Stage II: Carcinoma has involved the subvaginal tissue but has not extended to the pelvic wall	
Stage III: Carcinoma has extended to the pelvic wall	
Stage IV: Regional/distant spread excluding bullous edema	
IV A	Tumor invades the bladder and/or rectal mucosa and/or direct extension beyond the true pelvis
IV B	Spread to distant organs

10. Cancer statistics worldwide (GLOBOCAN 2020):

Indices	Males	Females	Both sexes
Number of new cancer cases	10,065,305	09,227,484	19,292,789
Age-standardized incidence rate	222.0	186.0	201.0

Contd...

Contd...

Indices	Males	Females	Both sexes
Risk of developing cancer before the age of 75 years	22.6%	18.6%	20.4%
Number of cancer deaths	05,528,810	04,429,323	09,958,133
Age-standardized mortality rate	120.8	84.2	100.7
Risk of dying from cancer before the age of 75 years	12.6%	8.9%	10.7%
5-year prevalent cases	24,828,480	25,721,807	50,550,287
Top five cancers	<ul><li>Lung, prostate, colorectum, and stomach</li><li>Liver</li></ul>	<ul><li>Breast, colorectum, and lung</li><li>Cervix uteri</li><li>Thyroid</li></ul>	<ul><li>Breast, lung, colorectum, andprostate</li><li>Stomach</li></ul>

11. Cancer statistics India (GLOBOCAN 2020):

Indices	Males	Females	Both sexes
Number of new cancer cases	646,030	678,383	1,324,413
Age-standardized incidence rate	95.7	99.3	97.1
Risk of developing cancer before the age of 75 years	10.4%	10.5%	10.4%
Number of cancer deaths	438,297	413,381	851,678
Age-standardized mortality rate	65.4	61.0	63.1
Risk of dying from cancer before the age of 75 years	7.4%	6.7%	7.1%
5-year prevalent cases	1,208,835	1,511,416	2,720,251
Top five cancers	<ul><li>Lip, oral cavity lung</li><li>Stomach</li><li>Colorectum esophagus</li></ul>	<ul><li>Breast and cervix uteri ovary</li><li>Lip and oral cavity</li><li>Colorectum</li></ul>	<ul><li>Breast</li><li>Lip, oral cavity, cervix uteri, and lung</li><li>Colorectum</li></ul>

12. **Gyne-oncology statistics worldwide (GLOBOCAN 2020):**

Cancer site	New cases				Deaths			
	Number	Rank	(%)	Cumulative risk	Number	Rank	(%)	Cumulative risk
Cervix uteri	604,127	8	3.1	1.39	341,831	9	3.4	0.82
Corpus uteri	417,367	16	2.2	1.05	97,370	20	0.98	0.22
Ovary	313,959	19	1.6	0.73	207,252	15	2.1	0.49
Vulva	45,240	31	0.23	0.09	17,427	31	0.18	0.03
Vagina	17,908	35	0.09	0.04	7,995	35	0.08	0.02

13. **Gyne-oncology statistics India (GLOBOCAN 2020):**

Cancer site	New cases				Deaths			
	Number	Rank	(%)	Cumulative risk	Number	Rank	(%)	Cumulative risk
Cervix uteri	123,907	3	9.4	2.01	77,348	2	9.1	1.30
Corpus uteri	16,413	22	1.2	0.29	6,385	23	0.75	0.11
Ovary	45,701	8	3.5	0.74	32,077	9	3.8	0.57
Vulva	3,447	33	0.26	0.06	1,694	32	0.20	0.03
Vagina	5,518	29	0.42	0.09	2,723	30	0.32	0.05

Recent Advances and Controversies in Gynecological Cancer

VULVAL CANCER

- Increase incidence of both vulvar intraepithelial neoplasia and invasive vulvar cancer in young women. This rising trend has been attributed to smoking, human papilloma virus (HPV) infection, and changing sexual behavior.[1]
- New category of HPV negative vulval cancer with *NOTCH1* and *HRAS* mutations and along with normal p53 expression. It has got intermediate prognosis.[2]
- Smaller surgical margin (5 mm) in sexually sensitive areas and urethral/anal margin may be an acceptable option. Clitoral sparing modified radical vulvectomy has been possible with good oncological clearance in selected cases.[3,4]
- Lymphatic-venous anastomosis to decrease the surgical morbidity arising from the inguinofemoral lymphadenectomy.[5,6]
- GROINSS-V III (the GROningen INternational Study on Sentinel nodes in Vulvar cancer III) to investigate whether the efficacy of treatment can be increased by enhancing the dose of radiotherapy and by adding concurrent chemotherapy to inguinofemoral radiotherapy.
- Testing for mismatch repair/microsatellite instability, *PD-1* and/or *NTRK* gene fusion in recurrent/progressive/metastatic disease.
- New International Federation of Gynecology and Obstetrics (FIGO) (2021) staging for vulval cancer **(Table 1)**[7]

CERVIX CANCER

- In sentinel lymph node negative cases, omission of parametrectomy in Stage I B 1 cervical cancer was evaluated in a study. But, the sentinel lymph node does not represent the requisite pelvic lymph node basin and that parametrectomy is always an essential component especially in larger sized tumors. Tailored surgery as per sentinel lymph node biopsy is a controversial topic and consensus as yet not evolved so far.[8-10]
- Revisiting surgical assessment by extending para-aortic lymphadenectomy in radical hysterectomy has shown no survival advantage in a recent study.[11]

Table 1: Staging for vulval cancer [International Federation of Gynecology and Obstetrics (FIGO) 2021]

Stage I: Tumor confined to the vulva and/or perineum and with negative nodes Depth of invasion is measured from the basement membrane of the deepest, adjacent, dysplastic, tumor-free rete ridge (or nearest dysplastic rete peg) to the deepest point of invasion.	
I A	Lesions ≤ 2 cm and stromal invasion ≤ 1 mm
I B	Lesions > 2 cm or stromal invasion > 1 mm
Stage II: Tumor of any size with extension to lower 1/3rd urethra, lower 1/3rd vagina, lower 1/3rd anus with negative nodes	
Stage III: Tumor of any size with extension to the upper part of adjacent perineal structures, or with any number of nonfixed and nonulcerated lymph node	
III A	Tumor of any size with disease extension to upper 2/3rds of urethra, upper 2/3rds of vagina, bladder mucosa, rectal mucosa, or regional lymph node metastasis ≤ 5 mm
III B	Regional (inguinal and femoral) lymph node metastasis > 5 mm
III C	Regional (inguinal and femoral) lymph node metastasis with extra-capsular spread
Stage IV: Tumor of any size fixed to bone, or fixed, ulcerated lymph node metastasis, or distant metastasis	
IV A	Disease fixed to pelvic bone, or fixed or ulcerated regional (inguinal and femoral) lymph node metastasis
IV B	Distant metastasis

Source: Olawaiye AB, Cotler J, Cuello MA, Bhatla N, Okamoto A, Wilailak S, et al. FIGO staging for carcinoma of the vulva: 2021 Revision. Int J Gynecol Obstet. 2021;155:43-7.

- Role of therapeutic lymphadenectomy offering survival advantage has been shown in early staged cervical cancer.[12]
- Current consensus is not recommending minimally invasive radical hysterectomy in early-staged cervical cancer as it has been associated with lower rates of disease-free survival and overall survival than open abdominal radical hysterectomy.[13]
- OUTBACK trial concluded that adjuvant chemoradiation given after standard cisplatin-based concurrent chemoradiation for women with locally advanced cancer cervix did not improve the overall survival or progression free survival.[14]
- EMBRACE trial to assess the clinical outcome of the image-guided radiotherapy in cervix. It includes RetroEMBRACE, EMBRACE I, and ongoing EMBRACE II. Recurrences, morbidity, and quality of life (QoL) after radiotherapy are the parameters that are addressed in EMBRACE I. While EMBRACE II uses the MRI-guided adaptive intensity-modulated radiotherapy (IMRT) for external beam radiotherapy (EBRT) with

simultaneously integrated boost for the nodes and MRI-guided adaptive brachytherapy with intensification by the interstitial brachytherapy needles. The scope of the study also extends to translational research by integrating evolving imaging modalities and biomarkers. Results of EMBRACE I showed MRI-based image-guided brachytherapy to be an effective modality of treatment in all stages of locally advanced cervical cancer.[15]

- Conjugated monoclonal antibodies (*Tisotumab vedotin*) are latest in the field of oncologic therapeutics and a phase II study in persistent, recurrent, and metastatic cervical cancer has been carried out with promising median overall survival of 8.3 months.
- Triapine (*Ribonucleotide reductase inhibitors*) in combination with platinum-based concurrent chemotherapy has been tested in a phase II trial with good outcome.[16,17]

ENDOMETRIAL CANCER

- It is a known fact that well-differentiated early-staged endometrial cancers are being seen in young women having polycystic ovarian disease. Use of levonorgestrel-releasing intrauterine contraceptive device (LNG-IUS) in such subset of patients provides a possible role with 75% overall response at 6 months of use. It has the advantage of lower side-effects with respect to weight gain and venous thromboembolism when compared to oral progestins. However, there is a possibility of having sanctuary sites in the myometrium with the use of LNG-IUS. A recent study showed 85.7% complete response rate at 3 months after a hysteroscopic resection followed by the use of LNG-IUS.[18-21]
- Sentinel lymph node biopsy in endometrial cancer will not identify metastases in 3% of patients with node-positive disease.[22,23]
- There has been some growing evidence of use of metformin in endometrial cancer. Decreased insulin sensitivity of the body tissues results in elevated levels of circulating insulin (increased insulin resistance). Subsequently, excessive insulin downregulates sex hormone binding globulin levels and upregulates estrogen and androgen levels in the blood. Thus, insulin resistance leads to an increased risk for endometrial cancer. Metformin (insulin sensitizer) promotes utilization of insulin by the body tissues and thus reduces the circulating levels of insulin. Metformin also suppresses endometrial cancer cell growth via cell cycle arrest, concomitant autophagy and apoptosis by inhibition of the *LKB1-AMPK-mTOR, PI3K-Akt,* and *IGF-1*-associated pathways.[24,25]

UTERINE SARCOMA

- *Loss of MMR, good prognostic marker of leiomyosarcoma*: Tumor diameter < 10 cm, mitotic index < 20/10 HPF and Ki67 negative.

- CDKN2A mutations and BRCA-2 mutations have been observed recently in leiomyosarcoma.[26-28]

OVARIAN CANCER

- Current recommendations offer testing for *BRCA-1* and *BRCA-2* mutations in all nonmucinous epithelial ovarian, Fallopian tube or peritoneal cancers. There is better overall survival in *BRCA* mutation patients due to better response to platinum-based chemotherapy.[29]
- Two recent trials validated similar overall survival outcomes with either neoadjuvant chemotherapy (NACT)/interval debulking surgery (IDS) or upfront primary debulking surgery (PDS) in epithelial ovarian cancer. However, neoadjuvant chemotherapy has got lesser morbidity in case of patients with high tumor burden and poor performance status. These trials further accounted that quality of life has been better in the NACT/IDS arm than PDS arm and that NACT/IDS arm was found to be noninferior to the PDS arm.[30,31]
- Recently, secondary debulking surgery has been validated by a prospectively randomized surgical and superiority trial. It shows an overall survival benefit of debulking surgery in recurrent ovarian cancer and highlights the importance of complete resection in recurrent ovarian cancer.[32]
- There have been some new developments with regard to the use of polyadenosine diphosphate-ribose polymerase (PARP) inhibitor olaparib as maintenance therapy in newly diagnosed *BRCA* positive advanced ovarian cancer and in relapsed *BRCA* positive ovarian cancer. Trials have substantiated its use and found lower disease progression and higher disease-free survival rate in the olaparib users. Two trials have suggested addition of PARP inhibitors to other chemotherapeutic agents even in non-*BRCA* ovarian cancer patients. Thus, the use of maintenance PARP inhibitor following response to the first-line therapy is evolving as a standard of care in case of high-grade serous and endometroid ovarian cancer.[33-36]
- There is a potential use of combined PARP inhibitors along with immune checkpoint inhibitors (*PD-1 blockers*) in the coming days. Lastly, a phase III trial is underway regarding the use of immunotherapy like oregovomab in ovarian cancer after the success of a randomized phase II trial.[37]

REFERENCES

1. Akhtar Danesh N, Elit L, Lyton A. Trends in incidence and survival of women with invasive vulvar cancer in the United States and Canada: A population-based study. Gynecol Oncol. 2014;124:314-8.
2. Nooij LS, Ter Haar NT, Ruano D, Rakislova N, van Wezel T, Smit VTHBM, et al. Cancer Therapy: Clinical—Genomic Characterization of Vulvar (Pre)cancers

Identifies Distinct Molecular Subtypes with Prognostic Significance. Clin Cancer Res. 2017;23(22):6781-9.

3. Woelber L, Choschzick M, Eulenburg C, Hager M, Jaenicke F, Gieseking F, et al. Prognostic value of pathological resection margin distance in squamous cell cancer of the vulva. Ann Surg Oncol. 2011;18:3811-8.

4. Chan JK, Sugiyama V, Tajalli TR, Pham H, Gu M, Rutgers J, et al. Conservative clitoral preservation surgery in the treatment of vulvar squamous cell carcinoma. Gynecol Oncol. 2004;95:152-6.

5. Morotti M, Menada MV, Boccardo F, Ferrero S, Casabona F, Villa G, et al. Lymphedema microsurgical preventive healing approach for primary prevention of lower limb lymphedema after inguinofemoral lymphadenectomy for vulvar cancer. Int J Gynecol Cancer. 2013;23:769-74.

6. Boccardo F, Valenzano M, Costantini S, Casabona F, Morotti M, Sala P, et al. LYMPHA Technique to Prevent Secondary Lower Limb Lymphedema. Ann Surg Oncol. 2016;23(11):3558-63.

7. Olawaiye AB, Cotler J, Cuello MA, Bhatla N, Okamoto A, Wilailak S, et al. FIGO staging for carcinoma of the vulva: 2021 Revision. Int J Gynecol Obstet. 2021;155:43-7.

8. Cibula D, Mc Cluggage WG. Sentinel lymph node concept in cervical cancer: current limitations and unanswered questions. Gynecol Oncol. 2019;152:202-7.

9. Baiocchi G, de Brot L, Faloppa CC, Mantoan H, Duque MR, Badiglian-Filho L, et al. Is parametrectomy always necessary in early-stage cervical cancer? Gynecol Oncol. 2017;146:16-9.

10. Tseng JH, Aloisi A, Sonoda Y, Gardner GJ, Zivanovic O, Abu-Rustum NR, et al. Less versus more radical surgery in stage I B1 cervical cancer: a population-based study of long-term survival. Gynecol Oncol. 2018;150:44-9.

11. Del Carmen MG, Pareja R, Melamed A, Rodriguez J, Greer A, Clark RM, et al. Isolated para-aortic lymph node metastasis in FIGO stage I A2-IB2 carcinoma cervix: revisiting the role of surgical assessment. Gynecol Oncol. 2018;150:406-11.

12. Shah M, Lewin SN, Deutsch I, Burke WM, Sun X, Herzog TJ, et al. Therapeutic role of lymphadenectomy for cervical cancer. Cancer. 2011;117:310-7.

13. Ramirez PT, Frumovitz M, Pareja R, Lopez A, Vieira M, Ribeiro R, et al. Minimally Invasive versus Abdominal Radical Hysterectomy for Cervical Cancer. N Engl J Med. 2018;379(20):1895-905.

14. Mileshkin LR, Moore KN, Barnes E, Gebski V, Narayan K, Bradshaw N, et al. Adjuvant chemotherapy following chemoradiation as primary treatment for locally advanced cervical cancer compared to chemoradiation alone: The randomized phase III OUTBACK Trial (ANZGOG 0902, RTOG 1174, NRG 0274). J Clin Oncol. 2021.

15. Pötter R, Tanderup K, Schmid MP, Jürgenliemk-Schulz I, Haie-Meder C, Fokdal LU, et al. MRI-guided adaptive brachytherapy in locally advanced cervical cancer (EMBRACE-I): a multi-centre prospective cohort study. Lancet Oncol. 2021;22(4):538-47.

16. Regalado Porras GO, Chavez Nogueda J, Poitevin Chacon A. Chemotherapy and molecular therapy in cervical cancer. Rep Pract Oncol Radiother. 2018;23:533-9.

17. Popović-Bijelić A, Kowol CR, Lind ME, Luo J, Himo F, Enyedy EA, et al. Ribonucleotide reductase inhibition by metal complexes of Triapine: a combined experimental and theoretical study. J Inorg Biochem. 2011;105:1422-31.

18. Farhi DC, Nosanchuk J, Silberberg SG. Endometrial adenocarcinoma in women under 25 years of age. Obstet Gynecol. 1986;68:741-5.

19. Pal N, Broaddus RR, Urbauer DL, Balakrishnan N, Milbourne A, Schmeler KM, et al. Treatment of low-risk endometrial cancer and complex atypical hyperplasia with the levonorgestrel-releasing intrauterine device. Obstet Gynecol. 2018;131:109-16.

20. Dhar KK, NeedhiRajan T, Koslowski M, Woolas RP. Is levonorgestrel intrauterine system effective for treatment of early endometrial cancer? Report of four cases and review of literature. Gynecol Oncol. 2005;97:924-7.

21. Laurelli G, Falcone F, Gallo MS, Scala F, Losito S, Granata V, et al. Long-term oncologic and reproductive outcomes in young patients with early endometrial cancer conservatively treated: a prospective study and literature update. Int J Gynecol Cancer. 2016;26:1650-7.

22. Rossi EC, Kowalski LD, Scalici J, Cantrell L, Schuler K, Hanna RK, et al. A comparison of sentinel lymph node biopsy to lymphadenectomy for endometrial cancer staging (FIRES trial): a multi-centre prospective study. Lancet Oncol. 2017;18:384-92.

23. Geppert B, Lönnerfors C, Bollino M, Persson J. Sentinel lymph node biopsy in endometrial cancer-feasibility, safety and lymphatic complications. Gynecol Oncol. 2018;148:491-8.

24. Sivalingam VN, Kitson S, McVey R, Roberts C, Pemberton P, Gilmour K, et al. Measuring the biological effect of presurgical metformin treatment in endometrial cancer. Br J Cancer. 2016;114(3):281-9.]

25. Takahashi A, Kimura F, Yamanaka A, Takebayashi A, Kita N, Takahashi K, et al. Metformin impairs growth of endometrial cancer cells via cell cycle arrest and concomitant autophagy and apoptosis. Cancer Cell Int. 2014;14:53.

26. Elvin JA, Gay LM, Ort R, Shuluk J, Long J, Shelley L, et al. Clinical benefit in response to Palbociclib treatment in refractory uterine leiomyosarcomas with common CDKN2A alteration. Oncologist. 2017;22:416-21.

27. Seligson ND, Kautto EA, Passen EN, Stets C, Toland AE, Millis SZ, et al. *BRCA 1/2* functional loss defines a targetable subset in leiomyosarcoma. Oncologist. 2018;24:973-9.

28. Hoang LN, Ali RH, Lau S, Gilks CB, Lee CH. Immunohistochemical survey of mismatch repair protein expression in uterine sarcomas and carcinosarcomas. Int J Gynecol Pathol. 2014;33:483-91.

29. Xu K, Yang S, Zhao Y. Prognostic significance of BRCA mutations in ovarian cancer: an updated systematic review with meta-analysis. Oncotarget. 2017;8:285-302.

30. Kehoe S, Hook J, Nankivell M, Jayson GC, Kitchener H, Lopes T, et al. Primary chemotherapy versus primary surgery for newly diagnosed advanced ovarian cancer (CHORUS); an open-label, randomized, controlled, non-inferiority trial. Lancet. 2015;386(9990):249-57.

31. Fagotti A, Ferrandina MG, Vizzielli G, Pasciuto T, Fanfani F, Gallotta V, et al. Randomized trial of primary debulking surgery versus neoadjuvant chemotherapy for advanced epithelial ovarian cancer (SCORPION-NCT01461850). Int J Gynecol Cancer. 2020;30(11):1657-64.

32. Du Bois A, Vergote I, Ferron G, Reuss A, Meier W, Greggi S, et al. Randomized phase III study to evaluate the impact of secondary cytoreductive surgery in recurrent ovarian cancer: Final analysis of AGO DESKTOP III/ENGOT-ov20. J Clin Oncol. 2017;35:15.

33. Moore K, Colombo N, Scambia G, Kim BG, Oaknin A, Friedlander M, et al. Maintenance Olaparib in Patients with Newly Diagnosed Advanced Ovarian Cancer. N Engl J Med. 2018;379(26):2495-505.
34. Pujade-Lauraine E, Ledermann JA, Selle F, Gebski V, Penson RT, Oza AM, et al. Olaparib tablets as maintenance therapy in patients with platinum-sensitive, relapsed ovarian cancer and a BRCA 1/2 mutation (SOLO 2/ENGOT-Ov21): a double-blind, randomized, placebo-controlled, phase3 trial. Lancet Oncol. 2017;18(9):1274-84.
35. Ray-Coquard I, Pautier P, Pignata S, Pérol D, González-Martín A, Berger R, et al. Olaparib plus bevacizumab as first-line maintenance in ovarian cancer. N Engl J Med. 2019;381:2416-28.
36. Coleman RL, Flemming GF, Brady MF, Swisher EM, Steffensen KD, Friedlander M, et al. Veliparib with first-line chemotherapy and as maintenance therapy in ovarian cancer. N Engl J Med. 2019;381:2403-15.
37. Ferrandina G, Braly PS, Terranova C, Salutari V, Ricci C, Raspagliesi F, et al. A randomized phase II study assessing an optimized schedule of oregovomab anti-CA125 vaccination with carboplatin paclitaxel (CP) relative to CP alone in front-line treatment of optimally cytoreduced stage III/IV ovarian cancer (EOC). J Clin Oncol. 2017;35(15 Suppl):5536.

Psychology in Cancer Management—An Overview

Understanding the psychology of a patient and right communication skills are essential attributes for bonding and empowering our patients. This chapter aims to sum up the various stages of emotional turmoil in the patient and the treating doctor that predominates during cancer treatment. The color of the emotional impact changes during the various stages of the treatment. Mental health disorders among cancer patients are more prevalent than for patients with other chronic illness. Positive communication, tailored information, and guidance by the oncology team are essential components of optimal outcome. Emotion upheaval is expected to be there but acknowledging them is important for moving forward in a positive direction. Understanding patient's perceptive and priorities just cannot escape core management in oncology. Providing targeted information, implementing treatment that aligns with patient's expectations, decreasing fear and anxiety about the unknown, facilitating compliance, and improving quality of life are pillars of holistic medicine.

Screening for early diagnosis of cancer such as a Pap smear test or HPV (human papilloma virus) DNA test may at sometimes be a stressful situation for someone. Fear and anxiety while awaiting a screening result can lead to daily life disruptions in 30% women. Hence, it is important to provide necessary information to a patient before conducting a screening test to avoid confusion and to ensure compliance during follow-up. It is found that even a referral to a cancer specialist for consultation may give rise to anxiety and depression!

It is an ineluctable fact that stress of cancer diagnosis triggers psychological and behavioral changes in an individual. Patients are usually in a state of denial, anger, and frustration when first confronted with a diagnosis of cancer. Patients land up in an unforeseen situation! Communicating such bad news to any patient is not an easy task for the attending doctor. Also, communication of health information is difficult whenever patient experiences high levels of stress. Use of "SPIKES protocol" (Setting/Perception/Invitation/Knowledge/Emotion/Strategy and Summary) is helpful for good communication and it ensures participation of patient. It is of utmost importance to realize the fact that the first step in cancer treatment should be in the right direction. Hence, it is imperative for a compassionate and empathetic approach by the treating doctor.

Onco-workup is an assessment of the origin of the cancer, extent of the disease spread, type of the cancer, and thus the presumed stage of the disease. After this workup, each case is discussed in a tumor board and a plan of action is made by the consensus of the oncology team. Doctor can allay the fear and anxiety of the patient by empowering the patient with the relevant inputs from onco-workup. Nowadays, treatment is available for every cancer and that early staged cancer can rather be completely cured unlike other chronic illnesses.

Pretreatment anxiety, misinformation, confusion, fear, and anxiety are seen in 60% of patients prior to start of surgery, radiotherapy, or chemotherapy. Most of the concerns crop up from shared knowledge based upon other's experiences without proper validity or from online stuffs shared by those who had an unsuccessful treatment. Confusion and stress from complex health information, unknown hospital setting, and multiple new care providers cannot be ignored. In fact, depression, adjustment disorder, mood, and anxiety disorders can be seen in 25–30% of newly diagnosed cancer patients. Genesis of various such psychological issues in a cancer patient should be addressed by the oncology team.

Depression arises from life disruption and uncertainty about one's health and future activities. Anxiety about treatment, toxicities, and side effects from cancer treatment, fear of being left out, are common among the cancer patients. Anger from loss of childbearing capacity, early onset menopause, and loss of body image may lie dormant but mitigating patient's anger should be a part of our therapeutic approach. Guilt from concerns such as smoking, previous unprotected sexual activity and HPV infection, and unhealthy lifestyles should be delicately managed. Because of such diverse psychological impact of cancer, many such patients do not understand the shared information provided about cancer management and rather develop own misperceptions! Till the phase of acceptance and adjustment by the patient, the treating doctor should be supportive and put forward a balanced approach of hope and honesty. In fact, hope and honesty are not mutually exclusive.

Cancer treatment encompasses specific time zones within which a component of therapy needs to be administered. For example, initial surgery may be accompanied by adjuvant radiation or chemotherapy and they are being carried out in a scientific and systematic sequelae. Cancer management is primarily being followed in the lines of established guidelines, but it is also a constantly evolving field wherein new modalities and interventions are also incorporated through various trials. Effective and useful information regarding relevant treatment plan is to be delivered in a positive and sensitive way. This may be required to be repeated and delivered using multiple means such as pamphlets, booklets, e-mails, and personal interviews. It is pertinent to assess the patient's understanding of the given information. Retention and recall about a given information may be hampered due to anxiety or depression of the patient. Positive thinking such as seeking information and asking for social support by the patient is good indicator for coping up stress with a positive sense of mind.

Once the treatment is planned, patient should be informed about the intended actions to be carried out. Faith and trust build up a positive bonding and lead to successful outcome. As the treatment of cancer is a radical approach, counseling the patient about the complications and morbidity arising out of it should be discussed. Fertility-preserving surgery, sentinel lymph node biopsy, Enhanced Recovery After Surgery (ERAS) guidelines, and minimal invasive approach are making foothold in the treatment arena of cancer management. Nowadays, recovery after a radical surgery is faster due to finer techniques, enhanced training, better instruments, and enhanced postoperative care.

Postoperative pain and delayed recovery are seen more in patient having anxiety or depression from cancer diagnosis. Loss of reproductive capacity and impairment of body image or function (arising out of vulvar surgeries, shortening of vaginal length, vaginal dryness, dyspareunia, decreased sexual desire, premature menopause, decreased vulval and vaginal sensation, stomas, etc.) are various important management concerns that require delicate redressals. Restoration of sexual functions by using vaginal dilators, vaginal moisturizers, Kegel's pelvic floor exercises, and hormone replacement therapy may be offered. Positive interpersonal relationship can enhance self-esteem and body image of a cancer survivor.

Worldwide collaboration and cancer network are providing real time development of oncology team. Thus, the best available treatment for every cancer patient can readily be updated by oncology team. The transition period after completion of cancer treatment provides some sense of relief to the patient. However, fatiguability, sexual dysfunction, and sleep disturbances take time to recover in most of the patients. Post-treatment rehabilitation is an important issue and needs to be discussed beforehand with the patient and family members. It involves physical, emotional, spiritual, social, and professional rehabilitation. This can be achieved by regular value-based conversations about treatment plans and goals. The aim is to mitigate the conflict between expectation and outcome.

Alternate healing approaches such as yoga, personal sports of choice, healthy diet, and disciplined life can surely lead to positive mindset in normalization of daily life. It is usually seen that cancer survivors show greater positive attitudes toward life and evolve stronger interpersonnel relationships. But, about 15–30% cancer survivors still may have persistent anxiety or depressive events. Recurrence and progressive disease are more stressful periods but surprisingly patients are found to be more resilient, receptive, and with better clarity about the planned management. Best supportive care, behavioral and cognitive therapy, group therapy, and family therapy should be integrated from initiation of the cancer management.

Facilitating maximum autonomy and dignity of patient should be the framework of holistic cancer treatment.

There has been a great advancement in cancer care and early detection by screening has open up the opportunity of complete cure. With more recovery and better care, needs of cancer survivors are widening. To sum up, cancer management should include empowering patient with comprehensive assessment, clarification, delineation, elucidation, and shared decision making.

"May your choices reflect your hopes, not your fears."

—Nelson Mandela

SUGGESTED ASSESSMENT PARAMETERS

1. Patient Health Questionnaire Nine-Symptom Depression Scale and General Anxiety Disorder Scale
2. Patient Reported Outcomes Measurement Information System (PROMIS) for Depressive and Emotional Distress/Anxiety Scale
3. National Comprehensive Cancer Network (NCCN) Single-item Distress Thermometer
4. Female Sexual Function Index (FSFI)
5. PROMIS Sexual Function and Satisfaction Scale

Biostatistics and Epidemiology

1. Sensitivity of a test:

   a. Detects true positive
   b. Detects true negative
   c. Detects false positive
   d. Detects false negative

2. Specificity of a test:

   a. Detects true positive
   b. Detects true negative
   c. Detects false positive
   d. Detects false negative

3. Amount of previously unrecognized disease that is diagnosed as a result of the screening test is:

   a. Net value
   b. Yield
   c. Cumulative value
   d. New adjusted value

4. Epidemiological triad includes all, *except*:

   a. Environment
   b. Host
   c. Agent
   d. Time

5. Physical Quality of Life Index (PQLI) includes all indicators, *except*:

   a. Infant mortality
   b. Life expectancy at age one
   c. Literacy
   d. Per capita GNP

6. Human development index (HDI) includes all, *except*:

   a. Life expectancy index
   b. Social developmental index
   c. Education index
   d. Gross national income index

7. As per the Human Development Index; India ranks in the world at:

   a. 150
   b. 131
   c. 71
   d. 51

8. Action taken prior to the onset of disease is:

   a. Tertiary prevention
   b. Secondary prevention
   c. Primary prevention
   d. Primordial prevention

9. Action which halts the progress of the disease in its initial stage and prevents complications is:

   a. Primordial prevention
   b. Primary prevention
   c. Secondary prevention
   d. Tertiary prevention

10. Intervention in the late pathogenesis stage of the disease to prevent disabilities is:

a. Tertiary prevention
b. Secondary prevention
c. Primary prevention
d. Primordial prevention

11. Health education is main intervention of:

a. Tertiary prevention
b. Secondary prevention
c. Primary prevention
d. Primordial prevention

12. Percentage of death due to chronic noncommunicable disease in India is:

a. 30%
b. 40%
c. 50%
d. 60%

13. Cigarettes and other Tobacco Products Act (COPTA) of Government of India was passed in:

a. April 2001
b. April 2003
c. April 2006
d. April 2009

14. National Cancer Awareness Day is observed every year on:

a. Seventh November
b. Fourth February
c. First July
d. Seventh December

15. World Cancer Day is observed every year on:

a. Seventh November
b. Fourth February
c. First July
d. Seventh December

16. "Socratic method" of communication is:

a. One-way communication
b. Two-way communication
c. Verbal communication
d. Nonverbal communication

17. Statistical average includes all, *except*:

a. Mean
b. Mean deviation
c. Median
d. Mode

18. Statistical diagram used to depict central tendency and also tracks extreme observations is:

a. Box and whisker plot
b. Error bar diagram
c. Stem and leaf plot
d. Scatter diagram

19. Graphical representation showing confidence interval is:

a. Scatter diagram
b. Box and whisker plot
c. Error bar diagram
d. Stem and leaf plot

20. Graphical representation of meta-analysis of randomized control trials is:

a. Forest plot diagram
b. Inverse normal plot
c. Stem and leaf plot
d. Scatter diagram

21. When there is an association between disease and exposure is:

a. Odds ratio > 1
b. Odds ratio < 1
c. Odds ratio = 1
d. None of the above

22. Characteristics of a normal distribution curve includes all, *except*:

a. Bell-shaped curve
b. Mean, median, and mode coincides
c. Area under the curve is 1 or 100%
d. 95% of the total area is formed by mean ± 1 S.D.

23. The design effect (Deff) in case of stratified random sampling is:

a. Deff < 1
b. Deff > 1
c. Deff = 1
d. Deff = 0

24. The hypothesis which disagrees with the null hypothesis is:

a. True hypothesis
b. Opposite hypothesis
c. Complimentary hypothesis
d. Alternate hypothesis

25. Chances of incorrectly rejecting a true null hypothesis are known as:

a. Type I error
b. Type II error
c. Type A error
d. Type B error

26. Chances of incorrectly accepting a false null hypothesis are known as:

a. Type I error
b. Type II error
c. Type III error
d. Type IV error

27. Level of significance is known as:

a. Type I error
b. Type II error
c. Type A error
d. Type B error

28. Pearson's Chi-squared test includes all, *except*:

a. Large sample size
b. Approximate in accuracy
c. Contingency table of arbitrary dimension
d. Interpretation by odds ratio

29. Fischer's exact test includes all, *except*:

a. Large sample size
b. Exact accuracy
c. 2 × 2 contingency table ideally
d. Small sample size

30. Hypothesis test of the mean of one or two normally distributed populations is:

a. Student "t" test
b. Student "x" test
c. Student "y" test
d. Alpha test

31. Testing the difference between two paired proportions is:

a. McNemar test
b. Student t-test
c. Alpha test
d. Beta test

32. Univariate test that is based upon standard normal distribution is:

a. Z test
b. X test
c. Y test
d. T test

33. Analytical test used to compare more than two population means:

a. Student t-test
b. Analysis of variance (ANOVA)
c. Z test
d. P test

34. Statistically significant p value is:

a. <0.01
b. <0.005
c. <0.05
d. <0.5

35. Nonparametric test includes all, *except*:

a. Mann–Whitney test
b. Wilcoxon signed rank test
c. Kruskal-Wallis test
d. Student's "t" test

36. Nonparametric test to ascertain the consistent differences between two paired observations without normal distribution is:

a. Sign test
b. ANOVA
c. Z test
d. Y test

37. Appropriate nonparametric test to detect the differences between two independent sample populations when the sample is not uniformly distributed and is small size.

a. ANOVA
b. Independent t test
c. Mann–Whitney-Wilcoxon test
d. Kruskal–Wallis test

38. Appropriate nonparametric test to detect the differences between three or more independent sample populations when the sample is not uniformly distributed and is small size.

a. ANOVA
b. Independent t test
c. Mann–Whitney-Wilcoxon test
d. Kruskal–Wallis test

39. Safety, dose, and adverse effects of a drug metabolism in human is done in:

a. Phase I of clinical trials
b. Phase II of clinical trials
c. Phase III of clinical trials
d. Phase IV of clinical trials

40. **Drug efficacy and optimal dosing regimens are assessed in:**

a. Phase I of clinical trials
b. Phase II of clinical trials
c. Phase III of clinical trials
d. Phase IV of clinical trials

41. **Comparison of the new drug against the current standard treatment is done in:**

a. Phase I of clinical trials
b. Phase II of clinical trials
c. Phase III of clinical trials
d. Phase IV of clinical trials

42. **Use of drug in general population after the approval of regulatory body to validate its safety and efficacy is:**

a. Phase I of clinical trials
b. Phase II of clinical trials
c. Phase III of clinical trials
d. Phase IV of clinical trials

43. **When a test trial is conducted to determine a clinically significant difference between two interventions is:**

a. Superiority trial
b. Equivalence trial
c. Noninferiority trial
d. Inferiority trial

44. **When a test trial is conducted to determine whether the new interventions is neither worse nor better than the established intervention is:**

a. Superiority trial
b. Equivalence trial
c. Noninferiority trial
d. Inferiority trial

45. **When a test trial is conducted to determine whether the new interventions is not inferior to another established intervention is:**

a. Equivalence trial
b. Noninferiority trial
c. Inferiority trial
d. Superiority trial

ANSWERS KEY

1. a	2. b	3. b	4. d	5. d	6. b	7. b
8. c	9. c	10. a	11. d	12. d	13. b	14. a
15. b	16. b	17. b	18. a	19. c	20. a	21. a
22. d	23. a	24. d	25. a	26. b	27. a	28. d
29. a	30. a	31. a	32. a	33. b	34. c	35. d
36. a	37. c	38. d	39. a	40. b	41. c	42. d
43. a	44. b	45. b				

NOTES ON BIOSTATISTICS AND EPIDEMIOLOGY

- *Health research should be based upon FINER principles*: Feasibility, Interesting, Novelty, Ethical and Relevant.
- Levels of review in health research:
  - Scientific review (novelty and justification)
  - Ethical review (based upon principles of Autonomy, Justice, Beneficence, Non-maleficence)
  - Regulatory review (foreign involvement, intellectual property)
- Study designs in health research:
  - Qualitative studies
  - Observational studies
  - Retrospective studies
- *Broad objective*: Descriptive study frame work is to *estimate* while Analytical study frame work is to *determine.*
- Descriptive studies:
  - Case reports
  - Case series
  - Ecological studies (Group as a unit of analysis)
  - Cross-sectional studies (Disease burden)
- *Analytical studies:*
  - Cohort studies (Prospective/Ambispective/Retrospective) for *Relative Risk*
  - Case control studies for *Odds ratio*
- Experimental studies:
  - Randomized control trial
  - Non-randomized control trial
- Relative Risk (RR) = Incidence of disease in exposed / Incidence of disease in unexposed

  RR = 1 means exposure is not associated with the disease

  RR > 1 means exposure is positively associated with disease

  RR < 1 means exposure is negatively associated with disease

  Relative risk is also known as rate ratio or risk ratio
- Odds ratio = Odds that a case was exposed/Odds that a control was exposed

  Odds ratio = 1 means odds of exposure among cases and controls are same

  Odds ratio >1 means odds of exposure among the cases are higher than controls

  Odds ratio <1 means odds of exposure among cases are lower than controls
- *PICOT principles*: Used to refine a study research question and it stands for Population, Intervention, Comparison, Outcome and Time.

- Study population is the population to which the results of the study will be inferred
- Objectives of Epidemiological studies:
  - Internal validity (Obtain an accurate estimate of disease frequency and effect of exposure on health outcomes in study population).
  - External validity (Obtain an estimate that is generalizable to relevant target populations).
- Errors in a study:
  - Random errors (unknown sources- increasing sample size and precision can minimize it).
  - Systematic errors (bias related and can distort the study in one direction. Can be minimized by improving the study design).
  - Confounders affect the outcome and study variables. It can be minimized by a good study design.
  - Effect modifiers has the capacity to modify the relationship between the study variables and outcome by independently affecting the outcome. They should be eliminated by a good review of literature.
- Methods used in review of literature:
  - Information seeking
  - Information retrieval
  - Database searching by Boolean Query (and/or/not)
  - Critical appraisal
  - Indexing
  Pubmed search by identifying MeSH (medical subject headings) and use of filters.
- Data quality and data collection in health research is based upon the principles of:
  - Reliability
  - Accuracy
  - Validity
  - Precision
  Lines in a database represent records while columns represent variables.
- Data cleaning means detecting and removing errors from the data.
- Data dredging means misuse of data analysis to find patterns in data that can be presented as statistically significant.
- Data mining means finding possible relationship between known variables in a already collected data.
- Fabrication in research studies means the data are not generated from study in question and rather taken from some other study. Falsification in research studies means data were manipulated to produce the results.
- Prevalence (P) is a static measurement and it is the number of existing cases (old and new) in a defined population at a specified point of time. Incidence (I) is a dynamic measurement and it is the number of new cases in a given period in a specified population.

- Period Prevalence = (Fraction of prevalent cases at the beginning of time period + Fraction of incident cases that develop during the period)/Size of the population for the same time period
- Point Prevalence = Fraction of the observed cases at time 't'/Population size at time 't'
- *Cumulated Incidence (CI):* Also known as Attack Rate
  Fraction of new cases/Population at risk in the beginning $\times 10^n$
- Incidence Density (Incidence rate)
  Fraction of new cases/Total person-time of observation $\times 10^n$
- Prevalence = Incidence $\times$ Duration of the disease
- Case Fatality is expressed as a ratio or proportion and is defined as the number of deaths from a disease to the number of cases.
- Age-specific incidence or mortality is the number of new cancers or deaths that occur over a specified time among individuals of a particular age group divided by the total population in that same age group.
- Age-adjusted incidence or mortality is obtained by summing weighted averages of the incidence or mortality rates for each age stratum.
- Mean is the sum of all values divided by the total number of observed values.
- Median is the middle value.
- Mode is the value that occurs most frequently.
- Co-efficient of variation (CV)% = Standard deviation $\times$ 100/Mean. It measures the dispersion of data points around the mean.
- Inter-quartile range is defined as the interval between the upper quartile (Q3) value and the lower (Q1)
- *Phases in Clinical trials:*
  - Phase I (Healthy volunteers usually up to 50 numbers and assess safety/acceptability)
  - Phase II (Low risk population up to 100 to 500 numbers and aims to determine long-term safety/dose/schedule/efficacy indicators)
  - Phase III (High risk population up to 1000 numbers and looks for the effectiveness)
  - Phase IV (Community based up to population of $\geq$ 1000 and is used as a tool for post-marketing surveillance)
- *Null Hypothesis:* It is a hypothesis that states that there is no statistical significance between the two variables in the hypothesis. It is the hypothesis that the researcher is going to disapprove.
- Alternate hypothesis is the opposite of the null hypothesis.
- *Type I Error (α):* The probability of rejecting a null hypothesis when it is true. α is the significance level of a test. Confidence level $(1-\alpha)$ is the probability that an estimate of a population parameter is within certain specified limits of the true value.
- *Type II Error (β):* The probability of accepting a null hypothesis when it is false.

Power $(1-\beta)$ is the probability of correctly rejecting the null hypothesis when it is false and reflects the ability of a study to detect an actual effect. Precision is a measure of how close an estimate is to the true value of a population parameter.

Your Score after Self-Assessment

1 A B C D	11 A B C D	21 A B C D	31 A B C D	41 A B C D	51 A B C D	61 A B C D	71 A B C D	81 A B C D	91 A B C D
2 A B C D	12 A B C D	22 A B C D	32 A B C D	42 A B C D	52 A B C D	62 A B C D	72 A B C D	82 A B C D	92 A B C D
3 A B C D	13 A B C D	23 A B C D	33 A B C D	43 A B C D	53 A B C D	63 A B C D	73 A B C D	83 A B C D	93 A B C D
4 A B C D	14 A B C D	24 A B C D	34 A B C D	44 A B C D	54 A B C D	64 A B C D	74 A B C D	84 A B C D	94 A B C D
5 A B C D	15 A B C D	25 A B C D	35 A B C D	45 A B C D	55 A B C D	65 A B C D	75 A B C D	85 A B C D	95 A B C D
6 A B C D	16 A B C D	26 A B C D	36 A B C D	46 A B C D	56 A B C D	66 A B C D	76 A B C D	86 A B C D	96 A B C D
7 A B C D	17 A B C D	27 A B C D	37 A B C D	47 A B C D	57 A B C D	67 A B C D	77 A B C D	87 A B C D	97 A B C D
8 A B C D	18 A B C D	28 A B C D	38 A B C D	48 A B C D	58 A B C D	68 A B C D	78 A B C D	88 A B C D	98 A B C D
9 A B C D	19 A B C D	29 A B C D	39 A B C D	49 A B C D	59 A B C D	69 A B C D	79 A B C D	89 A B C D	99 A B C D
10 A B C D	20 A B C D	30 A B C D	40 A B C D	50 A B C D	60 A B C D	70 A B C D	80 A B C D	90 A B C D	100 A B C D

**Take a self-test prior to the start of your preparation as a take-off examination.

**After completion of a particular chapter, again you take your self-test examination and analyze the gap in knowledge. Go through these topics from the standard reference books given below.

**Also read the chapter as a whole especially about the current management protocols by going through the NCCN and ESGO guidelines (available free online).

**It is also important to know about the recent important trials mentioned along with relevant chapters.

**Question patterns are generally divided into easy 40%, moderate 40%, and tough 20%.

**Ideal preparation time should be intensive and dedicated study time of a period of 1 month.

M.Ch Gynecological Oncology Seats in India			
SL No.	**State**	**Institute**	**Seats**
1	Assam	Dr Bhubaneshwar Borooah Cancer Institute, Guwahati	Proposed seats 02
2	New Delhi	AIIMS, New Delhi	02
3	Gujarat	BJ Medical College, Ahmedabad	04
4	Karnataka	Kidwai Memorial Institute of Oncology, Bangalore	03
5	Karnataka	St. Johns Medical College, Bangalore	01
6	Kerala	Amrita Institute of Medical Sciences, Kochi	02
7	Kerala	Regional Cancer Centre, Thiruvananthapuram	02
8	Maharashtra	Tata Memorial Centre, Mumbai	02
9	Odisha	Acharya Harihar Regional Cancer Centre, Cuttack	02
10	Tamil Nadu	Christian Medical College, Vellore	02
11	Uttarakhand	AIIMS, Rishikesh	01

DNB Gynecological Oncology Seats in India			
SL No.	**State**	**Institute**	**Seats**
1	New Delhi	Rajiv Gandhi Cancer Institute andResearch Centre	02
2	Haryana	Fortis Memorial Research Institute Gurgaon	01
3	Kerala	Lakeshore Hospital and Research Centre, Kochi	01

SL No.	**State**	**Institute**	**Seats**
4	West Bengal	Tata Medical Centre, Kolkata	02
5	Karnataka	Sri Shankara Cancer Hospital and Research Centre, Bangalore	01
Various institutes also offer Fellowship in Gynecologic Oncology:			

Reference Books and Guidelines
William's Gynecology
Langman's Medical Embryology
Te Linde's Operative Gynecology
Berek and Novak's Gynecology
De Vita Cancer–Principles and Practice of Oncology
Berek and Hacker's Gynecologic Oncology
Richard R Barakat Principles and Practice of Gynecologic Oncology
Dennis Chi–The New Edition of Principles and Practice of Gynecologic Oncology

- The National Comprehensive Cancer Network (NCCN) Guidelines
- The European Society of Gynecological Oncology (ESGO) Guidelines

All the best to you: May these books inspire you to become the best gyneoncosurgeon!

EU GSPR Authorised Reprsentative
Logos Europe, 9 rue Nicolas Poussin
1700, La Rochelle, France
Phone: +33 (0) 6 67 93 73 78
E-mail: contact@logoseurope.eu

www.ingramcontent.com/pod-product-compliance
Ingram Content Group UK Ltd.
Pitfield, Milton Keynes, MK11 3LW, UK
UKHW051940150726
7214IPUK00020B/356